SUGAR DETOX

30 Day Sugar Detox Diet

BONUS! 30 Day Sugar Detox Cook Book and 30 Day Sugar Detox Meal Plan Included!

VALERIE CHILDS

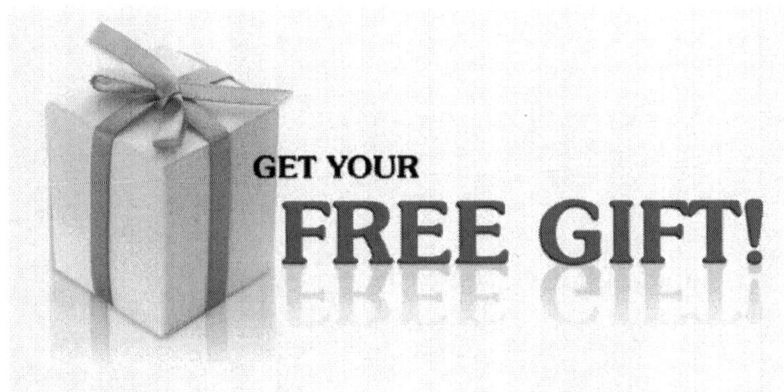

WAIT! – DO YOU LIKE FREE BOOKS?

My FREE Gift to You!! As a way to say Thank You for downloading my book, I'd like to offer you more FREE BOOKS! Each time we release a NEW book, we offer it first to a small number of people as a test - drive. Because of your commitment here in downloading my book, I'd love for you to be a part of this group. You can join easily here → **http://www.fatlosswithpaleo.com**

Bye, Bye, Sugar!
The Ultimate 30-Day Sugar Detox Guide

Table of Contents

Introduction

It doesn't matter if you've stumbled upon this book or if you've downloaded the book on purpose, I still want to congratulate you for taking the first step (or a step further) to a healthier "you" through sugar detoxing.

This book will teach you what sugar detox is all about and how it can help your body normalize its processes. It also contains a 30-day sugar detoxing guide, delicious and healthy recipes that you can try while on and after your detox, as well as helpful tips that will successfully usher you through the 30-day journey to a, possibly, sugar-free life.

Sugar-free? OK. I already feel some eyebrows rising. I understand that living a sugar-free life definitely sounds a little intimidating for many (*or for all of us*). Let's face it, sugar has been a part of our lives ever since we can remember – from the snacks that we ate as kids to the food we, now, consume as adults. We're used to putting sugar in our coffee, we're used to drinking sugary fruit juices and smoothies, we're used to eating sugary desserts and we're used to consuming sugary candy and candy bars, so it's as if sugar has been, and may always will be, a part of our lives and our diet.

We've been doing it for years and it does sound typical and harmless BUT, the problem lies in the amount of sugar we consume. We may not even know that the food we're eating already contains unhealthy amounts of sugar. We may not even be aware of the effects that it already has on our bodies.

As you read further into the book, I might be able to convince you that having sugar, especially too much sugar, spells trouble for your health and for the quality of your life. Are you ready to find out why? Then, as early as now, brace yourself because you're going to kiss that sugar goodbye! Let's get started!

Chapter 1

What is Sugar Detox?

What does Sugar Detox mean? Let's break down the term so we can understand it better:

1. **Sugar** – "a sweet crystalline substance obtained from various plants, especially sugar cane and sugar beet, consisting essentially of sucrose, and used as a sweetener in food and drink." *(Source: Google)*

2. **Detox** – is a shortened term for detoxification which is "a process or period of time in which one abstains from or rids the body of toxic or unhealthy substances." *(Source: Google)*

If we combine the two words together we get Sugar Detox which basically means abstaining from sugar for a period of time to eliminate it from one's body or to manage and control the intake of it. It is the process of allowing your body to get used to NOT getting as much sugar as it did before or NOT getting *any* sugar at all.

There are several sugar detoxing programs available in the market – 3 day sugar detox, 21 day sugar detox, 10 day sugar detox and so on – and each one has its own style and own guide to follow. Some programs will instruct you to go on a sugar fast for a number of days like 3 days and then allow you to eat a little bit of sugar after. Some programs will allow you to taper down the sugar in your diet gradually for a period of time. Some programs let you go cold turkey – yes, there are programs like this.

In particular, the Bye, Sugar Guide in this book gives you a 30-day guide to follow, complete with recipes, tips, motivation, and aftercare. This guide is focused on how you can clear your system of sugar with several healthy recipes to try out, with tips that can motivate you throughout your journey as well as with activities and other tips on what you can do after going through the Bye, Sugar Guide.

Chapter 2

ARE YOU UNCONSCIOUSLY ADDICTED TO SUGAR?

With all these talks about sugar and detoxing, you might be asking yourself the following questions:

- "Do I really need a sugar detox?"
- "Do I really need this Bye, Sugar Program?"
- "Why bother when I don't eat as much sweets as my friend or my father or my sweetheart?"
- "Why in the world would I need a sugar detox in the first place? I feel fine."

Let me tell you this: You're right to ask these kinds of questions.

It's normal to feel hesitation when faced with something new or something challenging but what we're going to do is to put things into perspective because, the truth is, most of us, if not all, are addicted to sugar and we don't even know it. It's an ugly truth but a truth nonetheless.

It may be surprising to hear that we're addicted to sugar unconsciously but it's actually possible that we are because we, going through our busy day and eating whatever works for us at that moment, aren't really conscious of the sugar content in the food we eat. Even if you say that you're not really eating a lot of "sweet stuff" it's still possible that you may be addicted.

Not convinced? To illustrate my point, I've compiled a short list of examples of surprising foods and drinks that have sugar in them. Check each item carefully and see what you're consuming on a daily basis:

Food / Beverage	Sugar (in grams & teaspoons)
Tomato based pasta sauce	15 grams (4 teaspoons)
Fat-free salad dressing	8 grams (2 teaspoons)
Commercially prepared smoothies	38 grams (9½ teaspoons)
Multi-grain cereals	6 grams (1½ teaspoons)
Multi-grain or whole-grain crackers	4 grams (1 teaspoon)
Barbecue sauce	12 grams (3 teaspoons)
Milk	12 grams (3 teaspoons)

Flavored yogurt	20 grams (5 teaspoons)
Energy bar	25 grams (6 teaspoons)
Red apple	20 grams (5 teaspoons)
Packed bread	6 grams per sandwich (1 ½ teaspoons)
Coleslaw	14 grams (3 ½ teaspoons)
Fruit drink	15 grams (4 teaspoons)
Coffee	30-60 grams (8-15 teaspoons)
Ketchup	6 grams (1 ½ teaspoons)
Sweetened tea	48 grams (12 teaspoons)
Coke	26 grams (6 ½ teaspoons)
Instant oatmeal	18 grams (4 ½ teaspoons)
Sports drink	20 grams (5 teaspoons)
Lemonade	25 grams (6 teaspoons)

(Disclaimer: the values may vary depending on the brand, the ingredients and the amount of food)

I bet you didn't expect some of the food that I included on the list. I, myself, was especially surprised with multi-grain cereals, whole-grain crackers, energy bars and packed bread. I wasn't expecting them to be on there and you probably didn't too. That's just how it is, though; some of the foods we eat actually have sugar in them without us knowing.

One way for us to be certain of sugar content in food is by checking the nutrition facts or the ingredients list at the back of the food packaging or by searching the internet for the amount of sugar per serving that's in a certain type of food. In short, we have to be conscious – sugar conscious.

Another way for us to tell if we've, indeed, consumed sugar, or too much of it, is by listening to our body. Our body always has clues that we need to decipher but most of the time, we rule signs out thinking that they're merely part of the body's natural process. It's time to change this way of thinking.

Review the following questions and answer them honestly. You may get a pen and a paper to write down the answers you have:

1. Do you consume certain types of food even if you you're not hungry at all?

2. Do you feel anxious when thinking about eliminating a certain type of food in your diet?

3. Do you feel tired or sluggish from over eating?

4. Do you consume food despite knowing and understanding the negative consequences?

5. Do you stress eat? Or eat to feel better emotionally?

6. Does eating a certain type of food make you euphoric?

7. Have you gone out of your house at wee hours of the night just to get a bite to eat?

8. Do you feel guilt after eating a certain type of food?

9. Do you routinely eat sweets when you're alone?

10. Do you experience physical symptoms when you go without sugar for a period of time?

Here's the verdict. If you answered YES to most or all of these questions, then you are addicted to sugar and it's a must for you to go on a sugar detox. You can't change what you already did in the past so don't feel guilty about it. The good news is, though we may not have known the kinds of foods that had unhealthy doses of sugar in them in the past, we can do something about it now, in the present, with the Bye, Sugar Program.

Chapter 3

WHAT SUGAR DOES TO US

Addicted to sugar or not, we still need to understand what sugar does to our body and we cannot do that without understanding the basics of the crystalline substance.

Common Types of Sugar Found in Food

Let's start here, with the common types of sugar that we can find in the food we eat. Knowing what these are will allow us to pinpoint what effect each one has on our bodies:

1. **Glucose** - Glucose is the main type of sugar in the blood and is the major source of energy for the body›s cells. Glucose comes from the foods we eat or the body can make it from other substances. Glucose is carried to the cells through the bloodstream. Several hormones, including insulin, control glucose levels in the blood. *(Source: Kids Health)*

Your body processes most carbohydrates you eat into glucose, either to be used immediately for energy or to be stored in muscle cells or the liver as glycogen for later use. Unlike fructose, insulin is secreted primarily in response to elevated blood concentrations of glucose, and insulin facilitates the entry of glucose into cells. *(Source: Healthy Eating SFGate)*

2. **Fructose** - is the principal sugar found in fruit. Humans don't produce fructose naturally and at high amounts, the substance could be deadly to our body – it can cause metabolic damage and it can trigger the early stages of diabetes and heart disease.

It is very different from other sugars because it has a different metabolic pathway and is not the preferred energy source for muscles or the brain. Fructose is only metabolized in the liver and relies on fructokinase to initiate metabolism. It is also more lipogenic, or fat-producing, than glucose which, primarily, the reason why it can cause or trigger the early stages of heart diseases as well as other. *(Source: Healthy Eating SFGate)*

3. **Sucrose** – commonly known as table sugar. It is a double sugar, containing one part each of glucose (50%) and fructose (50%), chemically bound together. Enzymes in the intestine quickly and efficiently split sucrose into glucose and fructose,

which are absorbed into the body as single sugars. *(Source: Food Insight)*

So, as you see, the types of sugars that require our main focus are glucose and fructose. They may have the same caloric value and they may be good sources of energy but they do have their disadvantages when taken in at dangerously high amounts.

Common Effects Sugar Has on Our Body

Let's zoom out from the cellular level and let's take a look at the effects of sugar on the body as a whole. Some of these are pretty common but some, as you'll soon found out, are pretty serious if you're sugar consumption is not taken control of. Let's get to it:

1. Destroys Teeth

This effect is pretty much common knowledge. Our dentists and our mothers have been telling us, ever since we were kids, to lay off the candy because it's going to ruin our teeth. That hasn't changed. Sugar is bad for the teeth because it provides easily digestible energy for the bad bacteria in the mouth. The result? Tooth decay and several agonizing visits to our family dentist.

2. Bad for the Liver

Many may not know this but sugar is broken down into 2 simple sugars before it enters the blood stream. These simple sugars are glucose and fructose *(see common types of sugar found in food)*. Let's focus on the latter – fructose. Fructose can only be metabolized by the liver in certain amounts.

It's no problem if we eat a little bit since the fructose will be turned into glycogen (for carbohydrate storage) and stored in the liver until the time comes that our body needs it. However, if the liver is full of glycogen, and if you're still taking in too much sugar, the liver will be forced to turn the fructose into fat to prevent the liver from overloading. Now, do you think would be the result for this one? Fatty liver, of course, and that may lead to a number of serious problems if left untreated. This includes:

- Cirrhosis
- Liver failure
- Liver cancer
- Liver-related death

3. Resistance of Insulin

Insulin plays an important role in our body's metabolism. Insulin's job is to regulate the metabolism of carbohydrates and fats by promoting the absorption of glucose from the blood to skeletal muscles and fat tissue and by causing fat to be stored rather than used for energy *(Source: Wikipedia)*. When insulin doesn't do what it's supposed to do, we can call this insulin resistance which can lead to metabolic syndrome, obesity, cardiovascular disease and type II diabetes.

4. Could Cause Cancer

Cancer is basically the uncontrolled growth and multiplication of cells in our body. Insulin is, actually, one key hormone that regulates this kind of growth. It is for this reason that many experts believe that having constantly elevated insulin levels can contribute to cancer.

So it's like cause and effect. Once you consume too much sugar, it could lead to insulin resistance. Once you have insulin resistance, it predisposes you to cancer. Consuming too much sugar may not be a direct cancer causer but studies have shown that people who eat a lot of sugar are at a much higher risk of getting the Big C.

5. Addiction & Dopamine

Sugar, as well as many other junk foods, triggers a massive dopamine release in our brain. Dopamine is a compound present in the body as a neurotransmitter and a precursor of other substances including epinephrine *(Source: Google)*. It is involved in movement, motivation, reward and addiction.

This is basically why sweets and junk foods are so addictive – they trigger a response in the reward center of our brain.

6. Contribute to Depression

It's true that eating sugary goodies can give you a temporary boost in your mood but overloading your system with sugar will eventually have the opposite effect. The exact mechanism of how sugar triggers a negative effect on your mood is actually unknown but some believe that insulin resistance may force the release of the stress hormones cortisol and GLP-1.

7. Increases the Risk of Yeast Infections

This one is particularly for the ladies. Yeast infections are usually caused by an overgrowth of Candida – bacteria that naturally exist in our body. These bacteria are usually under control thanks to the immune system but when your blood sugar is high, the excess sugars will also be found in your urine and saliva. These conditions are very conducive for the bacteria, Candida, to grow.

8. Brain Fog

If you've been having a hard time concentrating lately, it may be because of your sugar consumption or the high levels of sugar in your blood. "Research out of the University of California, Los Angeles, suggests that too much sugar forms free radicals in the brain and compromises nerve cells' ability to communicate" *(Source: Reader's Digest).* This will affect your memory, your thought process and your moods.

Wait There's More

These eight are already very good reasons on why we need to eliminate or cut down the sugar that we consume. However, we still need to remember that there are a lot more effects sugar has on our body – the list goes on. Other mention-worthy effects include: an increase in our waistline, heart disease and stroke (which are the no.1 cause of death for people with type 2 diabetes), it makes us hungry all the time and it makes us look older than we really are. All of these could be avoided just by cutting back or eliminating the sugar that you eat every day.

Chapter 4

The Benefits of Sugar Detoxing

Now that you know what sugar can do to our body, let's talk about what will happen when we successfully go through a sugar detox program. Yes, the list does go on when talking about sugar's harmful effects on our body but, the bright side is, the benefits of sugar detoxing are also almost endless.

The most obvious benefits are, of course, regaining your health and regaining control over your body. Specifically, though, I'd like you to wrap your mind around these 7 main sugar detoxing benefits:

1. Weight Loss

Even though weight loss isn't your main goal in doing a sugar detox, you'll still, most likely, be losing pounds because your body will have less sugar to turn into fat. Nonetheless, you still have to remember the most important thing: set realistic expectations.

Just because you know that weight loss is imminent while on a sugar detox, it doesn't mean that you're going to lose a lot of it. The weight loss that comes from sugar detoxing will not be dramatic but if you want better results in this department, losing more weight is possible if you pair this program with a good exercise routine.

2. Energy (that doesn't come from a sugar rush)

There's a reason why the expression called "sugar rush". You'll be in a "rush" with bursts of energy as soon as the sugar hits your blood stream but as soon as that sugar is gone, you'll also "rush" into feeling more tired than you felt before eating whatever sugary goodness you had on your hands.

Eliminating these bursts of energy from sugar will allow the natural energy from your body to take over. Imagine your day without having to reach for that extra cup of sugary coffee to perk you up. It may not be imaginable now but when the time comes, you'll be able to feel it and it's going to feel great!

3. Better Mood

With your natural energy flowing continuously throughout your body, a more positive mood will most likely follow. Studies have shown that cutting down sugar intake helps with anxiety and depression.

On top of that, you'll be eliminating your stress eating habit which also results to lesser feelings of guilt. How so? Well, when you stress eat, you feel guilty afterwards, right? Therefore, no stress eating equals to no guilty feeling.

An improved mood can bring about a lot of positive things in your life or even just in your day – you'll smile more, you'll be more productive and you'll feel like you can do anything you set your mind to. Who wouldn't want that?

4. Look Younger

A lot of people that went on sugar detox diets have mentioned an improvement on their skin or on their complexion. It has something to do with preventing Glycation – which is the binding of sugar and protein which damages on a cellular level. This is most evident on your skin. Preventing this will result in healthier and younger looking skin.

5. Concentration

Since sugar has been known to cause brain fog, eliminating it would result to the opposite. You'll be able to think clearly, you'll be able to concentrate more and you'll be able to get ideas quickly. Think of how productive your day will be if this happens!

6. Lesser Hunger Pains

Do you ever stop while in the middle of doing something because you feel hungry? Well, that's not going to happen when your body doesn't have the sugar that it's used to having to convert into energy.

Here's what happens: when you feed on sugar, your body mainly uses this as a source of energy. When you're all out of this energy source your brain is going to signal your stomach to start letting you know that it's time to refuel, like when your car runs out of gas. When your body's used to not having this kind of energy source, it will search for energy somewhere else like proteins or fat storage (yes, you heard that right, fat storage).

7. Prevention of Diseases

Last, but certainly not the least, you'll be preventing a number of diseases and you'll be taking yourself out of the list of people who are at high risk for these diseases. If you read the "What Sugar Does to Us" section thoroughly, you'll know that sugar can cause a lot of health problems. By simply detoxing yourself of this entails that you will prevent heart problems, stomach problems, insulin problems and so on that are caused by having too much sugar in your diet.

Now are you excited to get started with the program? Don't worry, we're almost there!

Chapter 5

Before Starting the Process

Before starting, there are a few things that you need to remember before embarking in this 30-day program. These reminders will help you set realistic expectations on how it will be and how you will feel when on the program.

1. It's going to be a challenge.

Breaking a habit is never easy. You really have to discipline yourself to stick to the program and keep at it for the duration of the time specified. There will be obstacles and temptations that you're going to face so you have to be prepared both mentally and physically.

Don't give up, though, because the harder the struggle the greater the victory. It's like climbing up a steep mountain, once you reach the top, you'll feel like your king or queen of the world.

2. Your patience will be stretched.

In every detox, you're going to deal with your body getting used to NOT having what it normally has had for years. Each person will have a different reaction to this but one thing is for sure your body will highly likely react negatively at first. Let's call it withdrawal – withdrawal from sugar.

As soon as this happens, you have to stretch your patience enough to get through this phase. Everything is going to be easier as soon as your withdrawal is over so you have to be patient enough to stick to the plan no matter how you feel.

3. You have to go in with a set goal or objective.

Every plan needs to have direction. For you to come out of this program successfully, you need to determine the direction of where this is going to lead you. If you're aiming to lose weight, make sure that you partner this guide with an appropriate exercise routine. If your goal is to eat healthier, make sure that you supplement this goal with organic produce, vitamins and etc.

You get the idea, right? What's your goal? Why do you need to do a sugar detox?

4. It might take longer than you think.

Your first sugar detox will, definitely, not be your last. Most people find it difficult to reset their body back to its natural state in just 30 days. You need not worry because you can do the sugar detox program for the second time or for the third time.

It really depends on how your body reacts to the program. If you've been a heavy sugar consumer then you might need to take a break after you do the program for the first time. After the break, you may opt to do the program for the second time and so on.

5. Adjust your lifestyle.

Here's another important thing to remember: this book is not a lifestyle guide. This book aims to educate and to guide you through meal planning but, ultimately, the lifestyle change will personally come from you. Go into this program thinking that you have to adjust your diet and your lifestyle so the approach is more holistic. You cannot have successful results without changing one or the other.

6. Keep things positive.

Always focus on the positive and never on the negative. The best way to do this would be to keep your eye on the prize rather than on the process. Before starting, the process may look intimidating – especially when it calls for you giving up coffee, cupcakes, cookies and whatnot. But if you look at it from the end, feeling happier because you look great, you have more energy and you're more productive, your mind won't perceive it as something that will be difficult to do.

Delve on these for a couple of days so you can have the right mind set upon starting the program. Bookmark this section and go back to it once you're ready to start.

Chapter 6

Bye, Sugar! 30 Day Sugar Detox Guide

Preparing for the Detox

Now for the fun part! The first step is always getting everything ready for the change that will happen. Aside from adapting the right mindset, you also need to go through the checklist below so you can optimize your sugar detox result through eliminating possible obstacles.

Prep Phase Checklist
Let your friends and family know about what you're doing. They are your support system so they have to know what's going on. Here are some things that you can tell your friends and family: 1. "I'll be going on a 30-day sugar detox journey so there will be some changes in my mood. If I seem grumpy, please lengthen your patience with me." 2. "It would be great if you could avoid consuming sugary snacks around me. It's going to make my process even more challenging."
Detox your kitchen first. Expect that you will have moments of weakness while on the program so you have to make sure that you cannot reach for something sugary. Eliminate all unhealthy snacks from your fridge, your pantry and wherever else you keep your secret stash of twinkies. Other food items that you can get rid of are processed food, gluten products, grain products, dairy products, refined or processed vegetable oil, alcohol products and any caffeine products.
Prepare a journal and a shopping checklist. A journal will let you jot down your emotions, write down encouraging phrases for you to read and, most importantly, it will allow you to document your progress. You can be as creative as you want with your journal. As for the checklist, you're going to need that so you won't forget anything when you go grocery shopping.

Wean off on sugar 2 days before the detox. Taper down your sugar intake 2 days before your detox. Cut your regular consumption of sugary or caffeinated items into half on the first day and then cut the half down to half on the second.
Measure your body and your weight. Weight loss may not be your number one goal but measuring yourself will help you track your progress. Before day 1 of the program, note down how much you weigh on your journal. You can also add your blood pressure on there. You can even add your starting waist line as well as measurements of your hips and thighs.
Prepare a blank calendar. It isn't enough to have a journal and a shopping checklist. You also need to have a blank calendar printed to serve as a visual reminder of what you're going to do (exercise for an hour, do grocery shopping, cook meals and so on) and what meal you're going to prepare and eat for the week. Since your calendar is going to be a visual reminder, put the calendar somewhere you can easily see it.

Calculate the calories that you need per day.

The calories that you need per day will depend on your current weight, gender and age. To calculate this you can refer to the chart below:

		Activity		
Gender	**Age**	Sedentary	Moderately Active	Active
Females	19 – 30	1800 – 2000	2000 – 2200	2400
	31 – 50	1800	2000	2200
	51 +	1600	1800	2000 – 2200
Males	19 – 30	2400	2600-2800	3000
	31 – 50	2200	2400-2600	2800-3000
	51 +	2000 – 2200	2200-2400	2400-2800

(Source: WebMD)

Calculating how much you need to consume to gain or lose weight is as simple as adding or subtracting 500. If you want to lose weight, deduct 500 to your total caloric intake for the day. If you need to gain weight, add 500 to your total. Doing this should make you gain or lose 1 pound per week.

Check the recipes and do your shopping and preparing a day before.

Preparation is the key to effortlessly going through each day of the 30-day guide. A day before you start, decide what you want to eat on your first week – what ingredients you need for the meals and snacks you need to prepare.

Write these down on your shopping checklist and then go shopping. Once you've bought everything, go to your kitchen and do the prepping for all of the meals and snacks for the first week. This is going to save you a lot of time, trust me.

Water is going to be your best friend. You're almost done with this checklist. The last thing that you need to prepare is your personal water bottle. Remember that water is going to be your best friend because you're going to drink lots of it while on the program. A personal water bottle (preferably with a measurement guide on the side) will be more convenient for you.

Once you have everything checked off, you're ready to begin!

Main Dishes

1. Parmesan Crusted Tilapia

Calories per Serving	Prep Time	Cook Time	Yields
203	10 mins	15 mins	3 Servings

Ingredients:

1/2 lb tilapia

2 tbsps olive oil

1/3 cup parmesan cheese

1 lime yields lime juice

Directions:

1. Preheat the oven to 450 °F or 230 °C.
2. While the oven is pre-heating, rinse and pat the fish dry using a paper towel. Sprinkle with your seasoning of choice.

3. Bake the fish in the oven for approximately 5 minutes.
4. In the meantime, mix the lime juice with the olive oil.
5. Take the fish out and drizzle the lime/oil mixture over it. Sprinkle the fish with parmesan cheese and put it under the broiler for 2 minutes or until the top of fish starts to brown.
6. Serve it while it's hot.

2. Dijon Broccoli Chicken

Calories per Serving	Prep Time	Cook Time	Yields
185	10 mins	30 mins	4 Servings

Ingredients:

- 1/2 cup chicken broth
- 1 tbsp soy sauce
- 4 cups flowerets broccoli
- 1 clove garlic, minced
- 1 tbsp olive oil
- 1 lb chicken breasts, cut into thin strips
- 6 tsps or 1 packet dijon mustard

Directions:

1. Mix the chicken broth and the soy sauce. Set it aside.
2. Cook the broccoli and garlic in hot oil over medium-high heat until crisp-tender. Remove from the broccoli from the

skillet and place it in another container. Cover it to keep it warm.

3. Add the chicken to the skillet. Cook and stir until cooked through.
4. Stir in your broth mixture. Bring your mix to a boil and then reduce the heat to medium-low. Stir in the mustard until it is well blended. Now you can mix the broccoli to the skillet.
5. Cook until heated through while stirring occasionally.
6. Serve and enjoy.

3. Salmon Burger Patties

Calories per Serving	Prep Time	Cook Time	Yields
223	10 mins	30 mins	4 Servings

Ingredients:

16 oz boneless salmon

3/4 cup panko Japanese style bread crumbs

1/2 medium red onion, diced

1 tbsp dijon mustard

1/2 tbsp canola mayonnaise

1 tbsp lemon juice

1/8 tsp cayenne pepper

1/8 tsp chili powder

1/8 tsp salt
1/8 tsp black pepper

Directions:

1. Preheat the oven to 375 °F or 190 °C. Lightly coat a baking sheet with cooking spray and set it aside.
2. Wash your hands thoroughly.
3. In a mixing bowl, use your hands to combine the salmon, bread crumbs, red onion, dijon mustard, mayonnaise, lemon juice, cayenne pepper, chili powder, salt, and pepper.
4. Take the mixture and shape it into 4 equally sized burger patties. Evenly space the patties on the baking sheet. Lightly spray the tops of the burger patties with cooking spray.
5. Bake for 25-30 minutes or until golden brown.
6. When burgers are cooked through, remove them from oven.
7. You may serve these patties on buns with toppings or you can also ditch the bun and just wrap the patties into some lettuce.

4. Coconut Chicken Tenders

Calories per Serving	Prep Time	Cook Time	Yields
240	10 mins	17-20 mins	6 Servings

Ingredients:

1.5 lbs boneless & skinless chicken breasts, cut into 20 tenders

2 large garlic cloves, crushed

1 + 1/4 tsp salt, divided

1/2 tsp ground black pepper

1 large egg

1 + 1/4 cup coconut flakes, unsweetened

1 tbsp garlic powder

1 tsp coconut oil

Directions:

1. In a medium bowl, add the chicken, the garlic, 1 tsp of salt and black pepper; mix and let marinate while you are getting other ingredients ready.
2. Preheat the oven to 425 ° F. Then, using your hands rub coconut oil on a large baking sheet.
3. In another medium bowl, lightly whisk the egg. In a large shallow dish, mix the coconut flakes, garlic powder and remaining 1/4 tsp salt thoroughly.

4. Dip each chicken tender in egg wash and then dredge in coconut flakes on both sides. Place each tender on the prepared baking sheet and repeat this step with the remaining chicken. If you run out of egg wash, you can either use another egg or just dredge in coconut flakes directly.

5. Bake for 17 minutes; flip the tenders and bake them for 5 more minutes or until a golden crust appears.

   NOTE: Ovens and baking sheets vary. The time guidelines provided are ideal for a light aluminum tray. Watch closely for the golden coconut flakes on the sides and bottom. Do not use parchment paper; it will take forever to cook.

6. Serve hot, as an appetizer or with a salad. You can make your own sauce, dip them in a bit of ketchup or enjoy them on their own.

5. Low Carb Mexican Rice

Calories per Serving	Prep Time	Cook Time	Yields
94	20 mins	20 mins	8 1-cup Servings

Ingredients:

1 large head of cauliflower (riced)

2 teaspoons olive oil

1 medium onion, minced

3 cloves garlic, minced

1 carrot, chopped

1 ear of corn, kernels cut off

½ cup fresh or frozen peas

1½ teaspoons sea salt

(could vary depending on your taste)

1½ teaspoons oregano

1 teaspoon cumin

1 teaspoon chili powder

1 teaspoon soya sauce

¼ cup tomato paste

2 limes

Directions:

1. Break apart the cauliflower, and "rice" half of it at a time in a food processor. Alternatively, you could finely chop it with a knife if you don't mind the process taking longer.
2. Add olive oil to a large wok or frying pan and saute the onions and garlic until they are soft over medium-high heat. Add the carrots, corn, and peas, and continue to saute the mix until the carrots are soft.
3. Add the spices and soy sauce to the vegetable mixture.
4. Add the riced cauliflower to the wok with the vegetable mixture, and add the tomato paste, stirring to lightly cover all of the "rice" mixture.

5. Continue to cook over medium-high heat for 8-12 minutes, until cauliflower is softened.
6. Garnish with fresh squeezes of lime juice and cilantro. These, of course, are just optional.
7. Serve and enjoy.

6. Grilled Rose Mary Salmon

Calories per Serving	Prep Time	Cook Time	Yields
186	5 mins	10 mins	4 Servings

Ingredients:

16 oz salmon

2 tsps extra virgin olive oil

1 fl oz lemon juice

1/4 tsp salt

1 dash pepper

2 cloves garlic, minced

2 tsps fresh rosemary, chopped

Directions:

1. Cut the fish into 4 equal-size portions.
2. Combine the olive oil, lemon juice, salt, pepper, garlic, and rosemary in a bowl. Brush the mixture onto the fish.

3. To grill, arrange the fish on a grill rack or use a grill basket sprayed with olive oil cooking spray.
4. Grill over medium-hot coals until the fish flakes easily

NOTE: Allow 4-6 minutes per 1/2" of thickness. If the fish is more than 1" thick, gently turn it halfway through grilling.

5. To broil, spray the rack of a broiler pan with olive oil cooking spray and arrange the fish on it.
6. Broil 4" from the heat for 4-6 minutes per 1/2" of thickness. If the fish is more than 1" thick, gently turn it halfway through broiling.
7. To serve, top the fish with capers, if using, and garnish with rosemary sprigs, if desired.

7. Grilled Chicken and Creamy Corn

Calories per Serving	Prep Time	Cook Time	Yields
267	12 mins	10-12 mins	4 Servings

Ingredients:

2 tablespoons olive oil

1 teaspoon smoked paprika

3 ears of corn, husks and silks removed

4 skinless, boneless chicken breast halves (1 to 1-1/4 pounds total)

1/4 teaspoon salt

1/8 teaspoon black pepper
1/3 cup light sour cream
Fat-free milk
1/4 cup shredded fresh basil

Directions:

1. In a small bowl, combine olive oil and paprika.
2. Brush the corn and chicken with your oil mixture. Sprinkle with salt and pepper.
3. For a charcoal grill, place corn and chicken on a rack directly over medium coals.
4. Grill, uncovered, for 12 to 15 minutes or until chicken is no longer pink. Turn it once.

NOTE: For a gas grill, preheat the grill. Reduce the heat to medium. Place the corn and chicken on grill rack over the heat. Cover and grill as above.

5. On a cutting board, place an ear of corn with the tip pointed down. While holding the corn firmly at stem end to keep in place, use a sharp knife to cut corn from the cob leaving some corn in planks.
6. Rotate the cob as needed to cut corn from all sides. Repeat with remaining ears.

NOTE: Use a kitchen towel to grip, if necessary.

7. Transfer corn to a bowl; stir in your sour cream. Stir in milk to desired creaminess. Slice chicken breasts. Serve with corn and sprinkle with shredded basil and then serve.

8. Marinated Flank Steak

Calories per Serving	Prep Time	Cook Time	Yields
302	5 mins	10 mins	4 Servings

Ingredients:

1 tsp cumin seed

3 cloves garlic

1/4 cup extra virgin olive oil

1 fl oz lime juice

1 tbsp red wine vinegar

1 tsp black peppercorns

16 oz flank steak

Directions:

1. Grind peppercorns and cumin seeds in mortar and pestle. Another option for grinding could be a coffee grinder. Or, you could just use pre-ground if you have too.
2. Combine the remaining ingredients in the blender. Blend well and pour over the flank steak in a ziploc bag.

3. Allow to marinate for at least 3 hours. **NOTE:** Much better if you leave it overnight.
4. Once you have your marinated flank ready, pre-heat the grill to medium-high heat. Oil the grate to prevent sticking.
5. Remove the meat from the marinade and discard the marinade and juices. Grill the meat for about 5 minutes per side, or until you achieve desired doneness.
6. Serve and enjoy.

NOTE: If you like your meat a bit on the rare side, try this method: Heat the grill to as high as it will go. Throw the meat on for 90-120 seconds. Flip and cook for another 90-120 seconds. Now turn off all the heat and allow the flank to cook for another 4-6 minutes. If your flank has a thicker middle; pound out the meat to a consistent thickness so that everything cooks to the same doneness.

9. Sweet Pepper Hash Brown Baked Eggs

Calories per Serving	Prep Time	Cook Time	Yields
179	10 mins	20-30 mins	8 Servings

Ingredients:

1 20 - ounce package of O'Brien-style refrigerated shredded hash brown potatoes

1 tablespoon olive oil

1 large green sweet pepper

1/2 cup pizza sauce

1/4 cup finely shredded Parmesan cheese (1 ounce)

8 eggs

Directions:

1. Preheat your oven to 375° F. Coat a 3-quart rectangular baking dish with cooking spray.
2. Add potatoes to prepared baking dish. Drizzle oil over potatoes; toss to combine.
3. Spread the potatoes evenly in the baking dish. Bake for 10 minutes. Stir the potatoes and then spread evenly in the baking dish again. Bake for 10 more minutes.
4. Meanwhile, slice the sweet green pepper into eight 1/4 to 1/2-inch-thick rings. Remove seeds. Remove potatoes from the oven. Reduce oven temperature to 350 ° F.
5. Arrange pepper rings in two rows on top of the potatoes. Spread 1 tablespoon of the pizza sauce within each pepper ring then break an egg into each pepper ring. Top each egg with a rounded teaspoon of the shredded Parmesan cheese.

Bake for 15 to 20 minutes more or until egg whites are set and yolks begin to thicken but are not hard.

6. Optional: If desired, garnish with freshly ground black pepper and/or snipped fresh basil.
7. Enjoy!

10. Bacon Wrapped Meatball

Calories per Serving	Prep Time	Cook Time	Yields
117	5 mins	35 mins	12 Servings

Ingredients:

1 lb ground beef

12 thin bacon slices

2 tsps garlic powder

2 tsps chili powder

1/4 tsp seasoned salt

1 medium egg

Directions:

1. Preheat the oven to 375 °F or 190 °C. Line a baking sheet with non-stick foil.
2. Mix all ingredients except bacon together in a mixing bowl.

3. Use melon a baller or something similar to create 12 medium sized meatballs.
4. Wrap each meatball in a slice of bacon.
5. Cook for 35 minutes.

11. Skinny Buffalo Chicken Strips

Calories per Serving	Prep Time	Cook Time	Yields
109	5 mins	10 mins	4 Servings

Ingredients:

1/2 tsp garlic powder

1/2 tsp paprika

1/2 tsp chili powder

1/8 tsp black pepper

1/4 cup red hot buffalo wing sauce

12 oz boneless skinless chicken breasts, cut into 8 strips

Directions:

1. Combine your garlic powder, paprika, chili powder and black pepper in a medium sized bowl. Season chicken with spices and toss evenly to coat the chicken.

2. Spray a large non-stick skillet with cooking spray and heat over medium-high heat. When hot add the chicken and cook until golden. This will take about 3-4 minutes. Turn the chicken over and cook it for another 3-4 minutes, or until center is no longer pink.
3. Pour the hot sauce over the chicken tossing it well.
4. Serve with celery sticks and blue cheese dressing if you like.

12. Thai Style Chicken Sausage

Calories per Serving	Prep Time	Cook Time	Yields
125	50 mins	10 mins	13 Servings

Ingredients:

40 oz boneless skinless chicken breasts

3/4 cup cilantro

2 tbsps less sodium soy sauce

2 tbsps ginger

2 tbsps garlic

juice of 1 lime

2 tbsps red curry paste

1 tsp coarse kosher salt

1/2 tsp black pepper

3 large egg whites

1 thick slice whole wheat bread

Directions:

1. Cut chicken into 1" cubes.
2. Mix remaining ingredients except egg whites and bread together well in shallow a dish or zip top bag.
3. Add chicken to marinade and place in freezer for 30 minutes.
4. Using food or meat grinder, fine disk grind the chicken and spices into a mixing bowl. Try to get all the chunks of garlic, cilantro, and ginger into the grinder. Grind the slice of bread last.
5. Using the flat beater or by hand mix in the egg whites. Stir about 3 minutes on "stir" or low or until the egg white is evenly distributed.
6. Form into 3 oz patties for grilling or pan frying in a bit of oil or drop it by half-teaspoonfuls into hot broth (boiling or simmering) for Asian style meatballs.

13. Pistachio Salmon Nuggets

Calories per Serving	Prep Time	Cook Time	Yields
74	50 mins	35 mins	10 Servings

Ingredients:

1 pound fresh or frozen skinless salmon fillets, about 1-inch thick

2 tablespoons water

2 tablespoons reduced-sodium soy sauce

1 tablespoon grated fresh ginger

2 teaspoons toasted sesame oil or cooking oil

1 tablespoon cooking oil

1 tablespoon finely chopped pistachio nuts

Directions:

1. Thaw fish, if frozen. Rinse fish and then pat dry with paper towels. Cut the fish into 1-inch chunks and then place the fish in a re-sealable plastic bag set in a shallow dish.
2. For marinade, in a small bowl, combine the water, soy sauce, ginger, and the 2 teaspoons sesame oil or cooking oil. Pour marinade over salmon chunks in bag. Seal the bag. Turn to

coat salmon. Marinate in the refrigerator for 30 minutes, turning bag occasionally.

3. Drain the salmon and discard the marinade. In a large nonstick skillet, heat the 1 tablespoon cooking oil over medium-high heat.

4. Add half of the salmon chunks to skillet; cook and gently stir for 3 to 5 minutes or until fish flakes easily with a fork. Remove from the skillet and place it on paper towels.

5. Cook and stir remaining fish; remove and place on paper towels. Transfer to a serving dish and sprinkle with pistachio nuts.

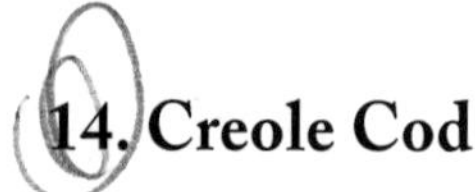

14. Creole Cod

Calories per Serving	Prep Time	Cook Time	Yields
148	10 mins	20 mins	4 Servings

Ingredients:

2 teaspoons olive oil

2 teaspoons Dijon mustard

1/2 teaspoon salt

1/2 teaspoon Creole seasoning blend (such as Spice Island)

4 (6-ounce) cod fillets (about 1 inch thick)

Cooking spray

1 tablespoon fresh lemon juice

Directions:

1. Preheat oven to 400°.
2. Combine first 4 ingredients; brush the mixture evenly over fish.
3. Place fish on a foil-lined baking sheet coated with cooking spray.
4. Bake at 400° for 17 minutes or until fish flakes easily when tested with a fork.
5. Drizzle juice evenly over fish; garnish with parsley, if desired.
6. Serve and enjoy.

15. Halibut Skewers

Calories per Serving	Prep Time	Cook Time	Yields
239	10 mins	20 mins	4 Servings

Ingredients:

1 1/2 pounds halibut, cut into 1-inch chunks

1 large red bell pepper, cut into 1-inch chunks

3 tablespoons prepared basil pesto

2 tablespoons white wine vinegar

1/2 teaspoon salt

Directions:

1. Preheat broiler.
2. Place the fish and the bell pepper in a shallow dish.
3. Drizzle pesto and vinegar over fish mixture; toss to coat.
4. Let fish mixture stand for 5 minutes.
5. Thread fish and pepper alternately onto each of 4 (12-inch) skewers; sprinkle evenly with salt.
6. Place skewers on a jelly-roll pan coated with cooking spray. Broil for 8 minutes or until desired degree of doneness, turning once.

16. Sirloin Steak with Deep Red Wine Reduction

Calories per Serving	Prep Time	Cook Time	Yields
162	15 mins	30 mins	4 Servings

Ingredients:

1/2 cup dry red wine

2 tablespoons balsamic vinegar

1 tablespoon reduced-sodium soy sauce

2 teaspoons instant coffee granules

2 teaspoons Worcestershire sauce

1/2 teaspoon coarsely ground black pepper

1 pound boneless beef sirloin steak, trimmed and cut about 3/4 inch thick

1/8 teaspoon salt

Nonstick cooking spray

Directions:

1. In a small bowl combine wine, vinegar, soy sauce, coffee granules, Worcestershire sauce, and pepper.
2. Place the steak in a large re-sealable plastic bag set in a shallow dish. Pour 1/4 cup of the wine mixture over the steak. Seal bag; turn to coat steak.
3. Marinate in the refrigerator 8 to 24 hours, turning occasionally. Stir the salt into the remaining wine mixture; cover and chill until needed.
4. Lightly coat a grill pan with cooking spray. Heat over medium-high heat. Drain steak, discarding marinade. Cook steak on hot grill pan 10 to 12 minutes or until desired doneness (145 degrees F for medium-rare), turning once halfway through cooking time. Transfer steak to a cutting board.

5. Let stand 3 minutes; thinly slice steak.

6. Meanwhile, in a small saucepan heat the reserved wine mixture to boiling over medium-high heat. Boil, uncovered, 2 to 3 minutes or until mixture is reduced to 1/4 cup.

7. Spoon wine mixture over sliced steak. If desired, serve with zucchini and/or sprinkle with oregano.

17. Orange and Rosemary Pork Chops

Calories per Serving	Prep Time	Cook Time	Yields
178	20 mins	30 mins	4 Servings

Ingredients:

4 4 - 5 - ounces boneless pork loin chops, cut 1 inch thick

2 teaspoons finely shredded orange peel

1/2 cup orange juice

2 tablespoons snipped fresh rosemary or 2 teaspoons dried rosemary, crushed

2 tablespoons Worcestershire-style marinade for chicken

1 tablespoon olive oil

1 tablespoon mild-flavor molasses or maple syrup

1/8 teaspoon ground black pepper

2 cups orange, apple, or peach wood chips or 6 orange, apple, or peach wood chunks

Directions:

1. Trim fat from chops. Place chops in a large re-sealable plastic bag set in a shallow dish.
2. For marinade: In a small bowl, combine orange peel, orange juice, the snipped or dried rosemary, Worcestershire-style marinade, olive oil, molasses, and pepper.
3. Pour marinade over chops. Seal bag; turn to coat chops. Marinate in the refrigerator for 4 to 24 hours, turning bag occasionally.
4. At least 1 hour before grilling, soak wood chips or chunks in enough water to cover. Drain before using. Drain chops, reserving marinade.
5. Arrange medium-hot coals around a drip pan. Test for medium heat above the pan. Sprinkle the drained wood chips or chunks over the coals. Place chops on the grill rack over drip pan. Cover and grill for 20 to 24 minutes or until pork is slightly pink in the center (160 degrees F), brushing once with marinade halfway through grilling. Discard any remaining marinade. If desired, garnish with rosemary sprigs. Makes 4 (4 1/2 ounces cooked meat) servings.
6. Enjoy!

18. Grilled Pork and Peach Salad

Calories per Serving	Prep Time	Cook Time	Yields
207	20 mins	25 mins	4 Servings

Ingredients:

1 pound pork tenderloin, trimmed and cut into 1-inch cubes

2 medium peaches or nectarines, pitted, and cut into 1-inch cubes

2 tablespoons honey

2 tablespoons orange juice

1 tablespoon low-sodium soy sauce

1/2 teaspoon curry powder

1/4 teaspoon ground black pepper

3 cups torn fresh Bibb lettuce

3 cups fresh baby spinach

1/4 cup bias-sliced green onions (2)

Directions:

1. On four 10-inch skewers, thread pork cubes. On three more 10-inch skewers, thread peach cubes.

2. For a charcoal grill, place skewers on the grill rack directly over medium coals. Grill, uncovered, for 8 to 10 minutes or until peaches are browned and for 10 to 12 minutes or just until pork is slightly pink in the center, turning occasionally.

NOTE: For a gas grill, preheat grill. Reduce heat to medium. Place skewers on grill rack over heat. Cover and grill as directed.

3. Meanwhile, in a large bowl stir together the honey, orange juice, soy sauce, curry powder, and pepper. When pork skewers are done, remove pork and peaches from skewers and place in honey mixture; toss to coat.

4. To serve, arrange lettuce and spinach on serving plates. Spoon pork and peaches evenly over greens. Sprinkle with green onions.

19. Sautéed Bass with Shiitake Mushroom Sauce

Calories per Serving	Prep Time	Cook Time	Yields
247	15 mins	10 mins	4 Servings

Ingredients:

2 teaspoons canola oil

1/8 teaspoon salt

1/8 teaspoon black pepper

4 (6-ounce) skinned bass fillets

2 cups sliced shiitake mushroom caps

1 teaspoon dark sesame oil

2 teaspoons bottled ground fresh ginger

1 teaspoon bottled minced garlic

1 cup chopped green onions

1/4 cup water

1/4 cup low-sodium soy sauce

1 tablespoon lemon juice

Directions:

1. Heat canola oil in a large nonstick skillet over medium-high heat.
2. Sprinkle salt and pepper over the fish. Add the fish to pan.
3. Cook for 2 1/2 minutes on each side or until fish flakes easily with a fork or until desired degree of doneness. Remove fish from pan; cover and keep warm.
4. Add mushrooms and sesame oil to pan; sauté 2 minutes. Add ginger and garlic to pan; sauté 1 minute.

5. Add the green onions and remaining ingredients to pan; sauté 2 minutes.

6. Serve with fish. Enjoy.

20. Pepper and Garlic-Crusted Tenderloin Steaks with Port Sauce

Calories per Serving	Prep Time	Cook Time	Yields
205	10 mins	15 mins	4 Servings

Ingredients:

2 teaspoons black peppercorns

1/2 teaspoon salt

3 garlic cloves, minced

4 (4-ounce) beef tenderloin steaks, trimmed (1 inch thick)

Cooking spray

1/4 cup port wine

1/4 cup canned beef broth

1 tablespoon chopped fresh thyme

Directions:

1. Place peppercorns in a small zip-top plastic bag; seal. Crush peppercorns using a meat mallet or small heavy skillet. Combine peppercorns, salt, and garlic in a bowl; rub evenly over steaks.
2. Heat a large nonstick skillet over medium-high heat. Coat pan with cooking spray.
3. Add steaks to pan. Reduce heat; cook 4 minutes on each side or until desired degree of doneness. Remove steaks from pan. Cover and keep warm.
4. Add port and broth to pan, stirring to loosen browned bits.
5. Cook until reduced to 1/4 cup (probably about 3 minutes).
6. Place 1 steak on each of 4 plates; drizzle each serving with 1 tablespoon sauce.
7. Sprinkle each serving with 3/4 teaspoon thyme.

Soup, Dressings, Salads

1. Blue Cheese Dressing

Calories per Serving	Prep Time	Cook Time
135	2 mins	2 mins

Ingredients:

1 cup regular mayonnaise (sugar-free)

1 cup sour cream

6 oz blue cheese

1 Tablespoon apple cider or wine vinegar

1/ 2 teaspoon pepper

Directions:

1. Crumble the blue cheese, and mix it all together.
2. Thin with water if desired.

2. Dijon-Lemon Vinaigrette Salad Dressing

Calories per Serving	Prep Time	Cook Time
25 per 1 tbsp	5 mins	5 mins

Ingredients:

3 tbsp water

2 tbsp lemon juice

2 tbsp extra-virgin olive oil

1 1/2 tbsp red wine vinegar

1 tbsp Dijon mustard

2 tsp minced garlic

2 tsp Worcestershire sauce

1/2 tsp fresh ground black pepper

1/4 tsp salt

Directions:

1. Combine all ingredients in a jar and cover tightly. Shake jar vigorously to mix ingredients well. Store in the refrigerator for up to one week.

3. Healthy Ranch Dressing

Calories per Serving	Prep Time	Cook Time
4 per 1 tbsp	5 mins	5 mins

Ingredients:

4 tablespoons freeze-dried parsley

1 1/4 teaspoons granulated garlic

1/2 teaspoon mustard powder

1/2 teaspoon onion powder

1/4 teaspoon dried thyme leaves dried

1/8 teaspoon dill weed

1/4 teaspoon fresh ground black pepper

1/4 teaspoon kosher salt

Directions:

1. Mix everything together and store in an air tight container.
2. Use 3 1/2 tablespoons per recipe of Ranch Dressing or use as a seasoning.

4. Carrot Ginger Dressing and Salad

Calories per Serving	Prep Time	Cook Time
158	5 mins	5 mins

Ingredients:

2 large carrots, peeled and roughly chopped

2 large shallots, peeled and roughly chopped

1/4 cup roughly chopped fresh ginger

2 tablespoons sweet white miso

1/4 tablespoon rice wine vinegar

2 tablespoons toasted sesame seed oil

1/2 cup grape-seed oil

1/4 cup water

1/2 teaspoon coarse salt

1/2 teaspoon freshly ground black pepper

1 head baby gem lettuce, roughly chopped

1/4 red onion, thinly sliced

1/4 avocado, diced

Directions:

1. Puree all the dressing ingredients together into a powerful blender until absolutely smooth.
2. Dress your salad, and enjoy!

5. Fresh Summer Corn Salad

Calories per Serving	Prep Time	Cook Time
124	5 mins	3 mins

Ingredients:

5 ears of corn, shucked

1/2 cup diced red onion

1 cup cherry tomatoes, halved

1 orange pepper, diced

1/2 cup fresh basil leaves, chopped

1 scallion, chopped

2 small jalapenos, seeds removed, chopped

2 tablespoons cider vinegar

2 tablespoons extra virgin olive oil

1/2 teaspoon salt

1/2 teaspoon pepper

1 tablespoon lime juice

Directions:

1. Place the corn in a pot of boiling salted water and cook for 3 minutes.
2. Drain and immerse in ice water.
3. Once cool, cut kernels off cob and place in serving bowl.
4. Add all other ingredients and enjoy or keep in refrigerator until ready to serve.

6. Miso Soup

Calories per Serving	Prep Time	Cook Time
60	3 mins	7 mins

Ingredients:

8 cups water

11/2 tsps dashi (instant, granules)

1/4 cup miso paste

1 tbsp seaweed (dried, for miso soup, soaked in water)

1/2 cup tofu (cubed)

2 tbsps green onions (chopped)

Directions:

1. Pour the water into a pot and bring to a boil. Add the instant dashi and whisk to dissolve. Turn the heat to medium-low and add the tofu. Drain the seaweed and add the seaweed to the pot. Simmer for 2 minutes.
2. In the meatime, Spoon the miso paste into a bowl. Ladle about 1/2 cup of the hot dashi broth into a bowl and whisk with chopsticks or a whisk to mix and melt the miso paste so that it becomes a smooth mixture.
3. Turn the heat off, add the miso paste to the pot and stir well. Taste the soup - if it needs more flavor, whisk in another tablespoon or two of miso paste. Top with green onions and serve immediately.

7. Miso Mushroom Soup

Calories per Serving	Prep Time	Cook Time
200	5 mins	15-20 mins

Ingredients:

1 qt vegetable stock

2 cups water

3 tbsps miso paste

14 ozs firm tofu (block of, cut in small cubes)

2 cups mushrooms (assorted, sliced or left whole if very small)

5 scallions

Directions:

1. Heat the stock and water to a simmer and add the mushrooms and tofu.
2. Simmer for a few minutes to cook the mushrooms.
3. When you're ready to serve, add the scallions and take off the heat. In a small bowl, whisk the miso with 1/4 cup of the hot broth to form a paste. Stir it back into the broth, and serve.

8. Pumpkin Soup

Calories per Serving	Prep Time	Cook Time
180	10 mins	50 mins

Ingredients:

2 tablespoons butter

2 celery ribs, diced

1 onion, chopped well

1 tablespoon flour

1 teaspoon salt

1/2 teaspoon ground ginger1

/4 teaspoon nutmeg

3 cups chicken stock

1 1/2 lbs diced pumpkin, roasted and peeled

1 cup half-and-halfchopped green onion

Directions:

1. Melt butter in large saucepan over medium heat. Add celery and onion and saute until onion is browned, about 10 minutes. Stir in the flour, salt, ginger and nutmeg. Cook for 5 minutes.
2. Stir in chicken stock and cubed pumpkin. Simmer on low for 30 minutes. Remove from heat and let cool for 10 minutes. Add to blender one cup at a time and blend until smooth. Add half and half and blend. Serve hot with green onion garnish.
3. Serve while hot!

9. Asparagus Soup

Calories per Serving	Prep Time	Cook Time
60	10 mins	10 mins

Ingredients:

1 white onion (small, 1/2-inch dice, 1 cup)

1 tbsp pure olive oil

1 carton vegetable stock (32oz)

1 lb asparagus (1-inch dice)

Salt and pepper

1/2 tsp herb seasoning salt

Directions:

1. Add onion and olive oil to stockpot on medium-low heat. Cook on low, stirring often for about 10 min, until onions are soft and translucent (but not browned).
2. Add stock and asparagus; season to taste with salt and pepper.
3. Bring to boil on high heat. Reduce heat and simmer for 5 mins, until asparagus is knife-tender.

10. Cream of Carrot

Calories per Serving	Prep Time	Cook Time
120	10 mins	20 mins

Ingredients:

2 tbsps butter

1 onions

6 carrots

1 liter vegetable stock

Salt and pepper

1 pinch thyme

Directions:

1. Slice the onion and cut the carrots into slices.
2. Put the butter and the onion in the pressure cooker and fry them lightly.
3. When the onion is transparent add the carrots. Fry lightly 1 or 2 minutes and stir it in the meantime.
4. Add the vegetable stock. Cook it for 15 minutes (It depends of your pressure cooker)
5. Carrots should be soft. Add the thyme and puree it.
6. Serve with some more thyme and grated cheese.

Breakfast Dishes

1. Sugar-Free Muffins

Calories per Serving	Prep Time	Cook Time	Yields
78	5 mins	8 mins	24 Servings

Ingredients:

1 cup any nut butter

2-3 ripe banana (preferable with tons of black spots)

2 eggs

1 teaspoon vanilla

10 drops liquid stevia, or a tablespoon or two of honey to taste (this is optional)

NOTE: The amount of stevia and honey will depend on your taste or how ripe your bananas are.

½ teaspoon baking soda

1 teaspoon apple cider vinegar

Directions:

1. Preheat oven to 400 degrees.
2. Place all ingredients into a blender or food processor.
3. Blend until well mixed. Watch out. The batter will be sticky!
4. Pour batter into a greased mini muffin tin.
5. Bake in a 400 degree oven for 8 minutes or so.
6. Serve and enjoy!

2. Hashbrown Breakfast Cups

Calories per Serving	Prep Time	Cook Time	Yields
140	5 mins	30 mins	4 Servings

Ingredients:

2 cups potatoes (shredded, from about 2 medium-sized potatoes)

1 egg whites

Salt and pepper

Parsley

2 eggs

Olive oil (for greasing)

Directions:

1. Preheat the oven to 440°F. In a bowl, mix together the shredded potatoes, egg white and salt, pepper and parsley to taste.
2. Grease two ramekins with the oil and divide the potato mixture evenly.
3. Using the back of a spoon, press the potato into the bottom of the ramekin and up the sides, creating a bowl. Bake in the oven for around 20 minutes or until golden brown.

4. Crack 1 egg into each of the potato bowls and return to the oven. Cook for a further 6 minutes if you want a drippy egg or 10 minutes if you want a solid yolk.

3. Crispy Egg Omelet

Calories per Serving	Prep Time	Cook Time	Yields
90	5 mins	15 mins	2 Servings

Ingredients:

4 eggs

1/4 bell pepper (diced)

1/4 roma tomatoes (diced)

1 mushrooms (diced)

Shredded cheddar cheese

1 green onion (sliced)

Directions:

1. Beat eggs in a mixing bowl. Stir in bell pepper, tomatoes, mushroom and mix.
2. Heat frying pan on medium heat and spread very little oil.
3. Pour a thin layer of the egg mixture on the pan.

4. After a few minutes when it seems sturdy enough, flip the omelet onto the other side in order to cook both sides.
5. Spread cheddar cheese on one half of the omelet and fold the other half over it.
6. After it reaches your desired level of cooked/crispy remove onto plate.
7. Garnish with green onions and enjoy

4. Breakfast Sausage or Patty

Calories per Serving	Prep Time	Cook Time	Yields
100	15 mins	25 mins	24 Servings

Ingredients:

1 lb ground pork

1 tsp sea salt (Celtic)

1 tsp sage

1 tsp thyme

1 tsp paprika

1 tsp black pepper

1/2 tsp cayenne pepper

1/2 tsp nutmeg

Directions:

1. Measure and mix spices.
2. Add spices to ground pork.
3. With hands, mix spices and pork together.
4. For mini-sausage balls, roll into 24 balls and place each one in mini-muffin tin.
5. Bake at 350°F for 20-23 minutes or until no longer pink in the center.
6. For sausage patties, form into 12 equal size patties.
7. Pan fry in cast iron skillet, on medium-high heat, 3-4 minutes per side or until no longer pink in the center.
8. Enjoy!

5. Veggie Frittata

Calories per Serving	Prep Time	Cook Time	Yields
110	15 mins	35 mins	8 Servings

Ingredients:

1 yellow onion (medium, chopped)

4 ozs fresh mushrooms (sliced)

1 tbsp olive oil

6 ozs baby spinach (fresh)

4 eggs (large)

6 egg whites (large)

1 cup reduced fat sharp cheddar cheese (shredded 2%)

1/4 cup grated parmesan cheese (freshly-)

2 tbsps fat free milk

1/4 tsp table salt

1/4 tsp nutmeg

Directions:

1. Preheat the oven to 350°. Sauté onion and mushrooms in hot oil in an ovenproof nonstick 10-inch skillet over medium-high heat 10 minutes or until tender.
2. Stir in spinach, and sauté 3 minutes or until water evaporates and spinach wilts.
3. Remove from heat, and set aside.
4. Whisk together eggs, egg whites, Cheddar cheese, and next 5 ingredients.
5. Pour egg mixture into skillet with onion the mixture, tirring to combine.
6. Bake at 350° for 12 to 15 minutes or just until set. Let stand 3 minutes.

7. Cut into 8 equal wedges.

8. Enjoy the wedges!

6. Cheesy Breakfast Muffin

Calories per Serving	Prep Time	Cook Time	Yields
63	10 mins	20 mins	12 Servings

Ingredients:

2 1/2 cups egg whites

3 eggs

3/4 cup reduced fat shredded cheese of choice

2 tablespoons of skim milk

Salt and pepper

Directions:

1. Preheat oven to 350 degrees F. Spray 12-cup muffin tin with nonstick cooking spray, you can also line with muffin tins, just make sure you spray the inside of the muffin tins.

2. Fill each muffin tin 1/4-1/3 full with veggies and herbs of choice.

3. Add in 1 tablespoon of cheese to each muffin tin.

4. In medium bowl whisk together egg whites, eggs, and milk. Fill each muffin to the top with egg mixture, pouring over the veggies already in each tin.
5. Bake for 20-30 minutes or until risen and slightly golden on top.
6. Let cool for a few minutes, then remove from tin.
7. Bon appetite!

7. Cheesy Spinach Baked Eggs

Calories per Serving	Prep Time	Cook Time	Yields
178	5 mins	15 mins	6 Servings

Ingredients:

4 teaspoons olive oil (divided in 2)

12 cups fresh spinach (divided in 2)

2 teaspoons minced garlic

1 cup shredded cheese of choice (use low fat version)

6 eggs

Directions:

1. Preheat your oven to 350 degrees.
2. Pour 2 teaspoons of oil in a large skillet.

3. Add 1 teaspoon of garlic and half the spinach.
4. Saute for 2-3 minutes until it is wilted.
5. Add 1/2 cup of cheese and stir until well combined.
6. Spray the ramekins with nonstick cooking spray.
7. Separate the spinach cheese mixture into 3 ramekins.
8. Add 2 more teaspoons of oil to your skillet, garlic and the rest of the spinach and cook as before.
9. Separate among 3 more ramekins.
10. Carefully crack one egg over each spinach mixture.
11. Bake for 15 minutes for slightly runny yolks.
12. Add some salt and pepper and some fruit.
13. Breakfast is served!

8. Bacon & Eggs B-fast Burrito

Calories per Serving	Prep Time	Cook Time	Yields
205	10 mins	10 mins	14 Servings

Ingredients:

12 slices turkey bacon

10 eggs

1/2 cup egg whites

1/2 cup milk, 1%

1 cup reduced fat shredded cheese

Directions:

1. Spray a large saute pan with nonstick cooking spray and cook your turkey bacon until crisp.
2. Set aside on paper towels. When cool chop into small bits.
3. In a bowl whisk together eggs, egg whites and milk.
4. Using the same saute pan, cook the egg mixture continuing to stir until scrambled.
5. Add cheese. Return bacon to pan and mix together. Cook until cheese is melted.
6. Lay tortilla on a piece of plastic wrap if making ahead or lay on a serving plate.
7. Scoop 1/3 cup of eggs and bacon in the middle of tortilla and fold up lengthwise, then each side and lengthwise again.
8. Wrap in plastic wrap then aluminum foil if freezing or store in fridge for up to 3 days.

9. Provencal Omelet

Calories per Serving	Prep Time	Cook Time	Yields
170	10 mins	20 mins	2 Servings

Ingredients:

Nonstick cooking spray

2 cups sliced fresh mushrooms

3 tablespoons sliced green onion

1 clove garlic, minced

1 cup refrigerated or frozen egg product, thawed, or 4 eggs

1/4 teaspoon herbes de Provence or dried thyme or basil, crushed

1/8 teaspoon salt

Dash ground black pepper

1 teaspoon olive oil

1/4 cup shredded part-skim mozzarella cheese (1 ounce)

1 tablespoon finely shredded Asiago or Parmesan cheese

1 medium plum tomato, chopped

Directions:

1. Lightly coat an unheated 6- to 7-inch nonstick skillet with flared sides with nonstick cooking spray. Preheat skillet over medium heat.
2. Add mushrooms, green onion, and garlic to skillet; cook until tender; stirring frequently. Remove mushroom mixture from skillet using a slotted spoon; set aside. If necessary, pour liquid out of skillet; carefully wipe out skillet.
3. In a medium bowl, combine egg product or eggs, herbes de Provence, salt, and pepper. Beat with a whisk or rotary beater until combined. Add 1/2 teaspoon of the oil to clean skillet. Preheat skillet over medium heat.
4. Pour half of the egg mixture into prepared skillet. Cook, without stirring, about 1 minute or until egg mixture begins to set. Run a spatula around edge of skillet, lifting egg mixture so uncooked portion flows underneath.
5. Continue cooking and lifting edges until egg mixture is set but is still glossy and moist. Sprinkle with half of the mozzarella cheese. Top with half of the mushroom mixture. Continue cooking until cheese just begins to melt.
6. Using the spatula, lift and fold an edge of the omelet partially over filling. Transfer omelet to a warm plate.

10. Poblano Tofu Scramble

Calories per Serving	Prep Time	Cook Time	Yields
182	10 mins	10 mins	4 Servings

Ingredients:

1 16 - 18 - ounce package extra-firm water-packed tofu (fresh bean curd)

1 tablespoon olive oil

1 -2 fresh poblano chile peppers, seeded and chopped (1/2 to 1 cup total)

1/2 cup chopped onion

2 cloves garlic, minced

1 teaspoon chili powder

1/2 teaspoon ground cumin

1/2 teaspoon dried oregano, crushed

1/4 teaspoon salt

1 tablespoon lime juice

2 plum tomatoes, seeded and chopped (about 1 cup)

Fresh cilantro sprigs (optional)

Directions:

1. Drain tofu; cut tofu in half and pat each half with paper towels until well dried. Crumble the tofu into a medium bowl. Set aside.
2. In a large nonstick skillet, heat olive oil over medium-high heat. Add chile peppers, onion, and garlic.
3. Cook and stir for 4 minutes. Add chili powder, cumin, oregano, and salt. Cook and stir for 30 seconds more.
4. Add crumbled tofu to chile pepper mixture. Reduce heat. Cook for 5 minutes, gently stirring occasionally. Just before serving, drizzle with lime juice and fold in tomatoes. If desired, garnish with fresh cilantro.

Side Dishes

1. Spinach with Garbanzo Beans

Calories per Serving	Prep Time	Cook Time	Yields
169	15 mins	10 mins	4 Servings

Ingredients:

1 tablespoon extra-virgin olive oil

4 cloves garlic, minced

1/2 onion, diced

1 (10 ounce) box frozen chopped spinach, thawed and drained well

1 (12 ounce) can garbanzo beans, drained

1/2 teaspoon cumin

1/2 teaspoon salt

Directions:

1. Heat the olive oil in a skillet over medium-low heat. Cook the garlic and onion in the oil until translucent, about 5 minutes.
2. Stir in the spinach, garbanzo beans, cumin, and salt. Use your stirring spoon to lightly mash the beans as the mixture cooks.
3. Allow to cook until thoroughly heated.

2. Zucchini Side

Calories per Serving	Prep Time	Cook Time	Yields
122	5 mins	5 mins	3 Servings

Ingredients:

3 zucchinis

1 sweet onion

2 tablespoons olive oil

Salt to taste

Directions:

1. Cut zucchini in half lengthwise, then slice crosswise into thin half-moons.
2. Cut onion into large dice.
3. Heat a large skillet over medium-high heat.
4. Pour in olive oil, then saute onion until lightly browned.
5. Stir in zucchini and continue to saute until zucchini is soft and lightly browned.
6. Season with salt to taste.

3. Green Beans with Lemon Juice

Calories per Serving	Prep Time	Cook Time	Yields
128	15 mins	5 mins	5 Servings

Ingredients:

1 clove garlic, peeled and cut in half

1/4 cup fresh lemon juice

1/4 cup olive oil

1 pound fresh green beans, trimmed

1 teaspoon salt

Directions:

1. Mix together the garlic, lemon juice, and olive oil in a large bowl; set aside.
2. Bring a large pot of salted water to a boil. Cook the green beans in the water for 5 to 6 minutes then drain.
3. Cool beans for about 10 minutes. Place cooled beans in the large bowl and toss with the lemon juice mixture; season with salt.
4. Allow beans to rest for 2 minutes before stirring again. Repeat 2 minutes rest and stirring once more.
5. Remove garlic before serving.

4. Mashed Sweet Potatoe

Calories per Serving	Prep Time	Cook Time	Yields
72	10 mins	20 mins	8 Servings

Ingredients:

3 sweet potato, peeled and cubed

1 butternut squash- peeled, seeded and cubed

1/2 teaspoon ground cinnamon

1/2 teaspoon nutmeg

1/4 cup sugar free maple flavored syrup

Directions:

1. Place the sweet potatoes and butternut squash into a large pot and cover with water. Bring to a boil over high heat, then reduce heat to medium-low, cover, and simmer until tender, about 20 minutes.
2. Drain and allow to steam dry for a minute or two.
3. Mash the sweet potatoes and butternut squash, then add cinnamon, nutmeg, and syrup.
4. Mix until smooth.
5. Serve with your favorite main dish.

5. Parmesan Chips

Calories per Serving	Prep Time	Cook Time	Yields
108	5 mins	5 mins	2 Servings

Ingredients:

1/2 cup parmesan cheese, grated

Directions:

1. Heat an 8" sauté pan over medium heat.
2. Sprinkle half the cheese evenly in the pan forming a "pancake".

3. Leave the "pancake" 2 to 3 minutes until melted and flip with a spatula.
4. Brown the second side.
5. Remove from pan to cutting board.
6. While still warm cut into triangles with a pizza cutter or sharp knife.
7. Repeat with remaining cheese.

6. Green Beans Alfredo

Calories per Serving	Prep Time	Cook Time	Yields
108	10 mins	30 mins	8 Servings

Ingredients:

16 oz green beans, frozen

6 oz cream cheese

16 fl oz cream

2 cloves garlic, minced

1 tbsp olive oil

3 oz shredded parmesan cheese (1 cup)

Directions:

1. Boil green beans in a quart of water until they start to get tender.
2. Drain green beans and place them in a medium baking dish. Set aside. Heat oven to 350 °F (175 °C).
3. In a saucepan, heat olive oil on medium heat.
4. Throw in minced garlic and stir until slightly browned, add heavy cream and cream cheese.
5. Break up cream cheese with spatula. Keep stirring until cream cheese is mostly melted. Remove from heat, stir in the parmesan cheese.
6. Pour cheese mixture over green beans and stir to coat.
7. Place in 350 °F oven for 20 minutes, stirring every 5 minutes.
8. Let cool about 10 minutes before serving.
9. Add in salt and pepper to taste.

7. Garlic Roasted Cauliflower

Calories per Serving	Prep Time	Cook Time	Yields
97	10 mins	60 mins	6 ½ Servings

Ingredients:

3 cups cauliflower florets

1/4 cup olive oil

1 tsp organic sea salt

1 tsp fresh milled black pepper

6 cloves minced garlic

1 Tbsp parsley

Directions:

1. Preheat oven to 400 degrees Fahrenheit.
2. Chop florets into small pieces. Toss with olive oil, salt, pepper, garlic and parsley.
3. Spread on a jelly roll pan and bake for 45-60 minutes, stirring every 15 minutes, until browned and crisp.
4. Makes 6, 1/2 cup servings. Store leftovers in the refrigerator, assuming there are leftovers.

8. Twice Baked Yams with Pumpkin

Calories per Serving	Prep Time	Cook Time	Yields
137	10 mins	60 mins	8 Servings

Ingredients:

8 small sweet potatoes

2 cups pumpkin

1 package cream cheese

Salt and pepper

Butter

Directions:

1. Preheat oven to 400 degrees.
2. Place yams on cookie sheet. Cut cross-hatch into the top (an "x") and bake for an hour. Let cool for 15 minutes.
3. Change oven temperature to 350 degrees.
4. Carefully peel back top edges from the yams.
5. Leaving the shells intact, scoop out the innards. Keep half and save the rest for another recipe. Mash yam innards. Add pumpkin, cream cheese and butter and mix until fluffy.
6. Spoon or pipe mixture back into the shells and bake for 20 minutes or until warm.

9. Au Gratin Turnips

Calories per Serving	Prep Time	Cook Time	Yields
178	15 mins	90 mins	8 Servings

Ingredients:

2 turnips (5" diameter), skinned, quartered and sliced thin

¼ cup chopped onion

2 Tbsp butter

2.5 cups cheese

½ cup heavy cream

½ cup organic chicken broth

1 tsp thickenthin/not starch

Salt and pepper to taste

Fresh chives (or dried) to taste

Grated Parmesan Cheese

Directions:

1. Place turnips in an ungreased 10" casserole.
2. Preheat oven to 325 degrees.
3. Over low heat, in a skillet, cook onion in butter until transparent (just a few minutes).
4. Add thickenthin/not starch, salt pepper and chicken broth just until boiling. Add cream and stir until heated.
5. Remove from heat and add cheese. Stir until cheese is melted and worked into the sauce.
6. Pour the thickened liquid over the turnips.

7. Bake for 1-1.5 hours or until turnips are tender. Sprinkle with ¼ cup Parmesan cheese mixed with ½ cup cheddar. Bake for 10-20 minutes more or until cheese has turned crusty.

10. Roasted Spaghetti Squash

Calories per Serving	Prep Time	Cook Time	Yields
137	5 mins	50 mins	4 Servings

Ingredients:

2 lbs spaghetti winter squash

2 tbsps extra virgin olive oil

1/2 tsp kosher salt

1/4 tsp black pepper

Directions:

1. Preheat oven to 425 °F (220 °C).
2. Cut squash in half, lengthwise.
3. Use a spoon to scrape out seeds and fibrous innards. Massage olive oil over the open halves and sprinkle evenly with the salt and pepper.
4. Roast, cut half up, on a foil-lined baking sheet for 40-50 minutes, just until the vegetable begins to take on a little light brown color.

5. Remove from oven and let cool until easily handled (about 30 minutes). Use a fork to gently scrape/pull the long strands away from the shell.
6. Use strands as the base to a cold salad or reheat in microwave, if necessary, and stir lightly with fresh parmesan cheese and basil chiffonade for a light side-dish.

NOTE: Roast squash on the weekend and you've got a go-to for a quick turn-around lunch or dinner.

Chapter 7

WHAT TO DO WHILE ON THE SUGAR DETOX

Here's where the program gets some structure. In this chapter, we will be talking about what you can do with all the information and the recipes that you've learned so far. You may be wondering why the structure came after the recipes.

Well, the answer is simple. Each person has a different eating habit that fits his or her daily routine. Each person also has a different daily caloric requirement which is based on his or her age and his or her level of activity (*see the checklist for a complete guide on daily calorie calculation*). In other words, not all persons are the same so we're going to show you how to customize this sugar detox plan to suit your lifestyle and your preferences.

Step 1

Go through the "Prep Phase Checklist" and make sure that you've done everything that's on that list.

Step 2

You should already know how much calories you would need per day. From this you will be doing a 4-week meal plan for yourself. There are no other guidelines except this: Discipline yourself. Stick to the plan and make sure you do not cheat.

Now, back to meal planning for 4 weeks. It's simple, really. All you have to do is to choose recipes that you'd want to try out for the day or for the week (*advance planning and advance preparation of meals are time savers, remember that*). These dishes have to equal your total calorie requirement for the day or for the week. You do the math and you do the planning. Here's an example of how you can do it:

Sample 1

DIET PROFILE
Gender: Female
Age: 27
Activity: Moderately Active
Sugar Detox Goal: Lose Weight and Eliminate Sugar from Diet *(this means that this person has to deduct 500 to her daily total calories)*
CALCULATION
2000 calories / day
- 500 for weight loss
1500 calories / day

WEEK 1

	Day 1		Day 2		Day 3	
	Dish	Calorie	Dish	Calorie	Dish	Calorie
Breakfast	Sugar-free muffins	78	Crispy Egg Omelet	90	Hashbrown Breakfast Cups	140
Lunch	Salmon Burger Patties Zuchini Side	223 122	Dijon Broccoli Chicken Miso Soup	185 60	Grilled Chicken and Creamy Corn	267
Snacks	Carrot Ginger Dressing and Salad	158	Water	0	Mashed Sweet Potatoe	72
Dinner	Parmesan Crusted Tilapia	203	Low Carb Mexican Rice Coconut Chicken Tenders	94 240	Marinated Flank Steak	302
Total Calories		**784**		**609**		**781**

WEEK 1 (Cont…)

	Day 4		Day 5		Day 6	
	Dish	Calorie	Dish	Calorie	Dish	Calorie
Breakfast	Veggie Frittata	110	Breakfast Sausage or Patty	100	Cheesy Spinach Baked Eggs	178
Lunch	Grilled Rose Mary Salmon	186	Skinny Buffalo Chicken Strips	109	Sweet Pepper Hash Brown Baked Eggs	179
Snacks	Salad with Blue Cheese Dressing	150	Asparagus Soup	60	Pumpkin Soup	180
Dinner	Halibut Skewers	239	Carrot Ginger Dressing and Salad Creole Cod	158 148	Dijon-Lemon Vinaigrette Salad Dressing Orange and Rosemary Pork Chops	200 178
Total Calories		**685**		**575**		**915**

WEEK 1 (Cont…)

	Day 7	
	Dish	Calorie
Breakfast	Bacon & Eggs B-fast Burrito	205
Lunch	Thai Style Chicken Sausage	125
Snacks	Healthy Ranch Dressing with Salad	140
Dinner	Sautéed Bass with Shiitake Mushroom Sauce	247
Total Calories		**717**

✓ Looking at each of the days in the sample meal plan for Week 1 tells us that you can have a day's worth of meals planned out but you still have room to eat some more. For example, the total calorie for Day 1 is 784. According to the sample calculation we did (*based on gender, age and activity level*), you still have 716 calories left.

✓ You can choose to look up other given recipes in this book to fill in the remaining calories or you can leave it as is to lose more weight.

Here's another way you can meal plan:

Sample 2

DIET PROFILE
Gender: Male
Age: 30
Activity: Sedentary
Sugar Detox Goal: Lose Weight and Eliminate Sugar from Diet *(this means that this person has to deduct 500 to her daily total calories)*
CALCULATION
2400 calories / day
- 500 for weight loss
1900 calories / day

WEEK 1

	Day 1		Day 2		Day 3	
	Dish	Calorie	Dish	Calorie	Dish	Calorie
Breakfast	Hashbrown Breakfast Cups Bacon & Eggs B-fast Burrito	140 205	Hashbrown Breakfast Cups Bacon & Eggs B-fast Burrito	140 205	Hashbrown Breakfast Cups Sugar-Free Muffins	140 x 3 servings = 420 78 x 3 servings = 234
Snacks	Whole Nuts (not in recipe)	200	Water	0	Water	0
Lunch	Asparagus Soup Salmon Burger Patties	60 223	Miso Soup Low Carb Mexican Rice Coconut Chicken Tenders	60 94 240	Grilled Chicken and Creamy Corn Mashed Sweet Potatoe	267 72
Snacks	Water	0	Whole-grain crackers, grapes, and cottage cheese	138	Water	0
Dinner	Carrot Ginger Dressing and Salad Parmesan Crusted Tilapia	158 203	Miso Soup Coconut Grilled Pork and Peach Salad	60 207	Miso Soup Marinated Flank Steak	60 302
Total Calories		**1189**		**1144**		**1355**

WEEK 1 (Cont…)

	Day 4		Day 5		Day 6	
	Dish	Calorie	Dish	Calorie	Dish	Calorie
Breakfast	Veggie Frittata Crispy Egg Omelet	110 x 2 servings = 220 90 x 2 servings= 180	Breakfast Sausage or Patty Crispy Egg Omelet	100 x 2 servings = 200 90 x 2 servings = 180	Cheesy Spinach Baked Eggs	178 x 2 servings = 356
Snacks	Water	0	Water	0	Water	0
Lunch	Grilled Rose Mary Salmon	186 x 2 servings = 372	Skinny Buffalo Chicken Strips Low Carb Mexican Rice	109 x 4 servings = 436 94	Sweet Pepper Hash Brown Baked Eggs Pumpkin Soup	179 180
Snacks	Water	0	Asparagus Soup	60	Home made popcorn (not in recipe)	40
Dinner	Salad with Blue Cheese Dressing Halibut Skewers	150 239 x 2 servings = 478	Carrot Ginger Dressing and Salad Creole Cod	158 148	Pumpkin Soup Orange and Rosemary Pork Chops Creole Cod	180 178 148
Total Calories		1400		1276		1461

WEEK 1 (Cont...)

	Day 7	
	Dish	Calorie
Breakfast	Bacon & Eggs B-fast Burrito	205 x 2 servings = 410
Snacks	Dijon-Lemon Vinaigrette Salad Dressing with Salad	250
Lunch	Thai Style Chicken Sausage Healthy Ranch Dressing with Salad	125 x 4 servings = 500 140
Snacks	Water	0
Dinner	Sautéed Bass with Shiitake Mushroom Sauce	247
Total Calories		1497

✓ Look at the calculations again for Sample 2. Not all calories were eaten up during each day so you still have room for more food or for more snacks.

- ✓ You can consume 2 or 3 or 4 servings of your favorite recipe as long as the calories do not exceed your requirement for the day.
- ✓ Since this program is flexible, you may snack on sugar free items such as nuts and then add in their calories to your daily calculation.

Sample 3

DIET PROFILE Gender: Female Age: 51 Activity: Sedentary Sugar Detox Goal: Maintain Weight and Eliminate Sugar from Diet (this means that this person has to stick to her daily total calories)
CALCULATION 1600 calories / day

WEEK 1

	Day 1		Day 2		Day 3	
	Dish	Calorie	Dish	Calorie	Dish	Calorie
Breakfast	Poblano Tofu Scramble Cheesy Spinach Baked Eggs	182 178	Provencal Omelet Cheesy Spinach Baked Eggs	180 178	Cheesy Spinach Baked Eggs	178 x 2 servings = 356
Snacks	Half of a Green Apple and cheese (not in recipe)	30 x 3 servings = 90	Pistachio nuts (not in recipe)	100	Veggies with Hummus Dip (not in recipe)	120
Lunch	Pepper and Garlic-Crusted Tenderloin Steaks with Port Sauce	205	Pepper and Garlic-Crusted Tenderloin Steaks with Port Sauce	205	Sautéed Bass with Shiitake Mushroom Sauce	247
Snacks	Water	0	Sugar free gelo (not in recipe)	10 x 3 servings = 30	Pistachio nuts (not in recipe)	100
Dinner	Sirloin Steak with Deep Red Wine Reduction Spinach with Garbanzo Beans	162 169	Sirloin Steak with Deep Red Wine Reduction Zucchini Side	162 122	Halibut Skewers	239 x 3 servings = 717

Total Calories		986		967		1540

WEEK 1 (Cont…)

	Day 4		Day 5		Day 6	
	Dish	Calorie	Dish	Calorie	Dish	Calorie
Breakfast	Veggie Frittata Sugar-Free Muffins	110 78 x 2 = 156	Sugar-Free Muffins Hashbrown Breakfast Cups	78 x 3 servings = 234 140 x 2 servings = 280	Hashbrown Breakfast Cups Crispy Egg Omelet	140 x 2 servings = 280 90 x 2 servings = 180
Snacks	Sun Flower Seeds (not in recipe)	120	Celery sticks and cream cheese (not in recipe)	80 x 2 servings = 160	Sugar free gelo (not in recipe)	10 x 2 = 20
Lunch	Grilled Pork and Peach Salad	207	Pistachio Salmon Nuggets Low carb Mexican Rice	74 x 5 servings = 370 94	Grilled Pork and Peach Salad	207
Snacks	Sun Flower Seeds (not in recipe)	120	Pistachio nuts (not in recipe)	100	Celery sticks and cream cheese (not in recipe)	80 x 3 servings = 240

Dinner	Creole Cod Parmesan Chips	148 x 3 servings = 444 108	Thai Style Chicken Sausage Green Beans Alfredo	125 x 2 = 250 108	Skinny Buffalo Chicken Strip Garlic Roasted Cauliflower	109 x 3 servings = 436 97
Total Calories		1256		1596		1460

WEEK 1 (Cont...)

	Day 7	
	Dish	Calorie
Breakfast	Crispy Egg Omelet Sugar-Free Muffins	90 x 3 servings = 270 78 x 2 servings = 156
Snacks	Sugar free gelo (not in recipe)	10 x 2 servings = 20
Lunch	Orange and Rosemary Pork Chops	178
Snacks	Rice cake with cheese (not in recipe)	85

Dinner	Bacon Wrapped Meatball Au Gratin Turnips	117 x 3 servings = 351 178
Total Calories		1238

- ✓ Let's look at the calculations in this sample. Did you notice anything? If you didn't, here's a clue: it has something to do with portions. Now, take a second look. One key to your sugar detox meal planning is portion management.
- ✓ Similar to the other meal plans I made, Sample 3 doesn't really consume the entire calorie requirement for the day. So, you can keep this as is or you can add a few more dishes to your diet.
- ✓ Remember that the program is flexible is if you're the kind of person that snacks in between meals, you can go ahead and research different sugar free snacks that you can munch on.

Things to Remember on Meal Planning:

- The first week, probably up to the second week, of sugar detoxing will be the most challenging. Make sure that you drink plenty of water whenever you feel the urge to eat something sugary.

- Do not deprive yourself. If you're used to eating snacks, that's no problem. Make sure that you incorporate something sugar-free and healthy in between meals. Sandwiches or wraps could be good snack choices.
- Plan your meals 3 days before your week starts. 2 days or 1 day before your week starts, you can begin shopping for your ingredients and begin prepping them (marinated, chopped, mixed and etc).
- I've already mentioned this on the prep phase checklist but no harm done in repeating this reminder: It will save you time to prepare your meals a day or two before.
- Stay within your calorie requirement. If you're snacking, make sure that you do your research on the different foods that are ok and not ok. I'm going to include a short list on this on the chapter.
- Make sure you adjust your calorie requirement according to your activity level. If you were sedentary and you began walking or jogging to go with your diet, you can move to moderately active. Adjust as you go so your body still gets the energy it needs.

- Here's another repeat reminder. Remember the blank calendar you're supposed to place somewhere in your kitchen you can easily see? Don't forget to fill it out and hang it.

Step 3

Your prep phase checklist is done and your meal planning is done. Step 3 is **water.** You may notice that the meal plans (*all three*) don't really have juice in them or coffee or smoothies. I designed it that way to make you drink more water.

Drinking water is a basic human need and there's no substitute for it. We can go several days without food but we won't be able to last a few days without water. This is because 60 or 70 percent of our body is made up of water. Slowly deplete that 60 or 70 percent and your body will cease to function.

Water is good for you and here are 10 reasons why:

1. It could help in weight loss.
2. It powers our warm-weather exercise.
3. It aids our digestion by helping the kidney and the liver flush waste products.
4. It protects against bladder cancer.
5. It could relieve headaches.

6. It helps make you feel energized as tiredness is a sign of dehydration.

7. It can help makes us more focused. Studies have shown that dehydration can make you lose your concentration more often.

8. It helps protect our joints and cartilages.

9. It takes the edge off hangovers.

10. It's been linked to heart health.

The benefits of drinking enough water in a day encompass 10. The bottom line is, drinking the right amount of water is good for you – both physically and mentally.

So how many glasses should we drink every day?

There are numerous opinions to this. However, health authorities commonly recommend following the 8x8 rule which states that we need to drink 8 x 8-ounce glasses of water (*2 liters or half a gallon of water*) on a daily basis. *(Source: Authority Nutrition)*

This applies when you're doing your daily routine like working, sitting in front of the computer, watching TV, reading a book and etc. You don't have to wait to feel thirsty to drink a glass of water.

This is primarily why it's a good idea to have your personal water bottle. You can keep track of the water you've already consumed and you can bring the water bottle with you anywhere you go; keeping it handy will make it easier for you to remember to drink water.

When you're working out, the amount of water that you're body will need is going to change. You'd need to increase the amount of water that you're consuming because you're also losing liquids through sweating.

IMPORTANT: Drinking plenty of water is healthy but drinking too much of it too fast could also lead to water toxicity.

Step 4

Your prep phase checklist is done and your meal planning is done. Your Step 3 is done. Now Step 4 has something to do with keeping you encouraged while on the 30 day program. Remember your journal? Here's what you need to write on it:

- ✓ For starters, write down your starting measurements and other starting metrics – fasting blood sugar, blood pressure, stomach girth and so on.
- ✓ Write down your daily caloric intake and then write down how you felt while on the meal plan for that day. Let's say your meal plan looks like this:

Day 1 Meals	Day 1 Calories
Hashbrown Breakfast Cups Crispy Egg Omelet	140 x 2 = 280 90 x 2servings = 180
Sugar free gelo (not in recipe)	10 x 2 = 20
Grilled Pork and Peach Salad	207
Celery sticks and cream cheese	80 x 3 = 240
Skinny Buffalo Chicken Strips Garlic Roasted Cauliflower	109 x 4 = 436 97

You can add tiny notes underneath the meals to describe what they taste like. It doesn't necessarily have to be the taste of every dish but notes that you'd want yourself to know or remember. For example:

Day 1 Meals	Day 1 Calories
Hashbrown Breakfast Cups Crispy Egg Omelet **NOTE:** Cook crispy eggs longer to make them crispier. They taste awesome! Consider cooking this again the next day.	140 x 2 servings = 280 90 x 2servings = 180 **NOTE:** Adjust servings. They're too small for your stomach!
Sugar free Gelatin **NOTE:** Gelo was alright but find an alternative sugar free snack.	10 x 2 = 20
Grilled Pork and Peach Salad **NOTE:** Family loved this dish. Need to cook for everyone on Friday.	207
Celery sticks and cream cheese **NOTE:** Fantastic snack!	80 x 3 = 240 **NOTE:** Eat more of this. Adjust calories.

Skinny Buffalo Chicken Strips Garlic Roasted Cauliflower **NOTE:** Too much garlic on the cauliflower. Lessen next time.	109 x 4 = 436 97

You can even add pictures if you like so you can appreciate the hard work that you've put into putting the meals together. You can be as creative with this as you like; don't be scared to use colored pens, strings, stickers and whatever designing materials you'd like to add.

The next things that you're going to put on your journal are words of encouragement for yourself. You can write down positive quotes or you can write down inspirational stories to keep you going. There are loads that you can find online. Here's a couple:

Inspirational and Motivational Quotes

> "It is better to take many small steps in the right direction than to make a great leap forward only to stumble backward."
>
> —Old Chinese Proverb

> "Whether you think you can or can't, you're right."
>
> —Henry Ford

> "The significant problems we face cannot be solved by the same level of thinking that created them."

—Albert Einstein

"We must be the change we wish to see in the world."

—Mahatma Gandhi

"When you blame others, you give up your power to change."

—Dr. Robert Anthony

"There are two primary choices in life: to accept conditions as they exist, or accept the responsibility for changing them."

—Dr. Denis Waitley

"Decide what you want, decide what you are willing to exchange for it. Establish your priorities and go to work."

—H. L. Hunt

"Confidence, like art, never comes from having all the answers; it comes from being open to all the questions."

—Earl Gray Stevens

"People may doubt what you say, but they will believe what you do."

—Lewis Cass

"Movement is a medicine for creating change in a person's physical, emotional, and mental states."

—Carol Welch

Links to Inspirational and Motivational Stories

- I Did It! Weight Loss Success Stories

- Get Inspired to Get Fit
- Shape Fit's Before and After (One of my favorites)
- Fast Diet Success Stories
- The Best Weight Loss Stories

Step 5 (Optional)

Your motivation is now on track! Step 5 is actually optional because this step needs for you to decide on the exercise routine you want to do while on a diet. Again, I'm telling you that this is optional especially if you just want to eliminate sugar from your diet. But, if you want to lose weight (*like a lot of it*), I strongly suggest adapting a work out plan. It doesn't have to be a full body work out too. It can be a 30 min run through your nearest park. It could also be a 30 minute walk around your block. The choice is up to you.

Step 6

Measure yourself again – blood pressure, waist, arms, legs, blood sugar, etc – and decide on your post sugar detox plan. Then, start preparing for it. Yes, you need to prepare for what you're going to do after your program because you've already put it too much work and you've already gone through a lot of progress. You do not want to waste these and go back to your old, nasty ways of eating a lot of sugar and unconsciously getting addicted to it.

There are three choices that you can make:

1. You could continue your sugar-free eating habit that you've, hopefully, coupled with a healthy lifestyle. (*The best choice out of the three*)
2. You could introduce small or healthy amounts of sugar into your diet and continue with your exercise routine. (*Second best choice you can m*ake)
3. You could go back to your old eating habits and lead a sedentary lifestyle. (*The absolute worst choice you could make*)

The choice is yours and to help you decide let's move on to the next chapter.

Chapter 8

What to Do After the Detox

Like what I said earlier, you have 3 choices. At this point, you may feel a little anxiety or fear about what's going to happen after – if you'll have the strength to continue or if you'll fail because you became lazy. It's normal to feel this way but remember this: you completed a 30-day guide so why not do 30 more days? Or even 90 more days?

Let me paint a clearer picture for you. Here's what's going to happen when you:

Live a Sugar Free Life

Because of the changes that you've already made while you were doing the 30-day sugar detox, a lot of things will have changed and are going to change. Your outlook and disposition will have changed to something more positive, your taste buds will have changed as well as your habits.

If you're really serious about going sugar free permanently, you're going to have to maintain these changes by:

1. Eating right.

- You have to make sure that no sugar goes into your food. This means that you have to make reading food labels a habit and/or sticking to foods that you can prepare from scratch. You have to make sure that whatever goes into your system does not have slight traces of sugar. This call for self-discipline and, sometimes, a strong will power to really make an effort into checking and preparing the food you eat.
- You have to permanently say goodbye to certain types of food.
- You may need to sacrifice during holidays and vacations.

2. Drinking right.

- So we've already had that long talk about drinking the right amount of water. You would have to remember to drink the right amount every day. You still have your personal water bottle so make use of it especially when measuring the amount of water you would need.

3. Thinking right.

- Aside from the will power that you're going to exert, you'd have to keep your journaling up so you stay motivated. If you're tired of writing on paper, a good idea would be to put up a blog and get your own sugar free weight loss story out there.

NOTE: Since you've already gone on this road before, not a lot of physical changes will occur. You can expect that the battle is going to be more mental because you will come across temptations and circumstances that may potentially make you fall off of the wagon.

Watch Your Sugar

Here's the second option. Re-introduce sugar (*healthy amounts of it*) in your diet. Depending on how you look at each choice, you may think that this one is easier but think again. Your body is going to adjust, little by little, to the amount of sugar that you're taking in even if they are in healthy doses.

Physical changes may include:

- A change in your digestive functions.
- Headaches may occur.

- A changed in your appetite.
- A changed in your energy level

Mental changes may include:

- A change in your mood.
- A change in your concentration.

When re-introducing certain types of food into your system, you have to take it 3 days at a time. This means that you would have to add 1 type of food and monitor the changes in your body for 3 days. Continue the process for each new food you eat like fruits. As much as possible, stay away from gluten containing foods and opt for vegetables, well-raised meat and eggs and naturally occurring fats.

A list of foods you need to re-introduce first:

- Fruit:
- Grass-fed dairy
- Dark chocolate
- Gluten-free grains or legumes
- Wine (*small amounts of it, like a glass*)

Very much like how you planned your meals when you were sugar detoxing, you would also need to plan your meals so you can gradually re-introduce the allowable types of food into your diet.

You can also take note of the changes that occurred like if you had a change in your energy while adding in yogurt or if you had headaches after drinking a glass of wine.

Go Back to Your Old Ways

This is the least of the choices you'd want to make. If you mentally decide to let everything go back to how they were before, you're not going to give a care about how much sugar you're consuming. The tendency is for you to go on a sugar binge which is bad for your body.

Going on a sugar binge will shock your system and you might experience severe physical reactions like headaches, mood swings, loss of energy and the like. Soon enough, you will experience the same sugar addict symptoms you had before your detox – brain fog, unstable digestion, always eating even if you weren't hungry. Those sound really unappealing!

I don't want you to go back to your old ways because you've come so far. You've already made the changes you wanted to make to be healthier, to be more energetic and to be more positive. It's highly likely that you're feeling good about yourself, you're concentrating better and you're more productive during the day. Why change your habits now when you've already formed new ones – better ones?

I encourage you to consciously make the decision to continue eating healthy and living healthy. You might think that this is just one compartment of your life and it won't affect the other compartments like your relationship, your success in your career and so on. But, I'm here to tell you that eating healthy and living healthy has loads to do with the other compartments.

Why, you ask? Because, all the other compartments have to have a base and that base is made up of: a healthy body, a healthy mind, and a healthy outlook. Continue eating and living right and see all the other things in your life follow.

Here are some inspiring people that have gone through a similar process as you did but have chosen to continue with either living sugar free or watching the sugar that they take in:

- A Hopeful Loser
- Real People's Comments
- Pilates 1901

You can look for more success stories online. Again, I want to tell you again that you're on your way to getting the "you" you've always wanted to have. Don't give it up for sugar!

Chapter 9

Making Your Detox a Success

As you may have imagined, going on a sugar detox is not easy because it requires you to adjust everything from your eating habits to your daily routine. You will struggle at first – that's a given – but there are ways to make that struggle more bearable. Here are tips that will help you make your sugar detox successful:

- **Eliminate soda** from your fridge and, ultimately, your diet. Soda is loaded with sugar and most of us are used to drinking one can per day. Replace this with water. Once you're drinking water often, even if you're just taking small sips at a time, you won't even be thinking of drinking half a can of soda.

- **Read labels.** I've already mentioned this before; you have to make reading labels a habit. It's essential that you do so because there are hidden sugar ingredients in some foods that may catch you off guard.

Here's a fan fact for you: There are more than 200 types of added sugars used in processed foods and beverages. Added sugars are used in more than 75% of the products sold in supermarkets – often, in unexpected items like bread, salty snacks and condiments.
(Source: Pop Sugar Infographic)

When reading the label, you have to watch out for those hidden sugars. If you see any one of the names listed below, it's best that you steer clear of the food product you're holding:

Sneaky Sugar Name	Commonly Found In (but not limited to)
Agave nectar (also known as agave syrup)	Cereals, Ice cream, Some organic foods
Barley malt	Malt beers, Cereals, Candy bars
Beet sugar	More than 20% of the worlds sugar
Blackstrap molasses	Baked beans, Ginger bread
Brown rice syrup (also known as rice syrup or rice malt)	Rice milk, Cereal bars, Some organic foods

Brown sugar	Baked goods, Beverages, Some sauces
Buttered sugar (also known as buttercream)	Cookies, Icing, Frosting
Cane juice crystals	Yogurt, Cake, Cookies, Baked goods
Cane juice	Used as a beverage, In liquor (Cachaça)
Cane sugar	80% of the world's sugar
Caramel	Sodas, Desserts, Candy
Carob Syrup	Cakes, Cookies, and used as a substitute for Chocolate
Corn Syrup	Sodas, Fast food, Cookies
Dextran	Used as a food additive
Ethyl maltol	Breads, Cakes, Confectionary goods
Galactose	Fast foods, Vegetable products, Dairy products
Golden sugar	Cake, Biscuits, Meringues
High fructose corn syrup	Fast foods, Sodas, Yogurts, Canned foods, Frozen pizzas, Macaroni and cheese, Cereal bars, Breads

Sorghum	Cereals, Cakes, Muffins, Beer, Other alcoholic beverages

Helpful links on How to Spot Sugar on Labels:

- Hungry for Change
- Huffington Post
- Low carbs diet
- Diabetes.org
- Healthy Eating

- **Go for fruit.** Yes, fruit contains sugar but it also contains fiber which helps slow down the processing of sugar in our bodies

- **Easy on the condiments**. In the earlier chapters of this book, we already talked about most condiments having loads of sugar. With this said it would greatly help your sugar free living or controlled sugar living if you ease up on the condiments or avoid them altogether.

- **Time your meals**. The idea here is to avoid making you feel too hungry. If you're as hungry as a tyrannosaurus rex, the tendency is to eat whatever is in front of you. It'll be great if you have something healthy in front of you but you still need to watch your portions and calculate your daily calorie requirement. The best choice for you would be to time your meals so it works with your daily routine.

- **Don't forget your journal.** This is why journaling whatever or however you feel is a requirement because this is going to be your motivator. Keep your motivations going by writing down positive things to yourself!

- **Also, don't forget water.** Another thing that you shouldn't forget: WATER. Keep your personal water bottle close and take small sips whenever you feel like eating something sugary.

- **Don't be afraid to modify the meal planning.** So we've already talked about how to go about constructing or planning your meals out for the week. You already have a guide but don't be afraid to modify it to whatever suites you. People who have inserted their personal touch on their sugar detox program have been found to have come out to be more successful in continuing their new sugar free habit.

- **Remember your goal.** You may lose sight of what you really want out of your sugar detoxing. This is where journaling comes in handy. If you did write down your goal(s) and starting measurements, you'll be able to go back to it anytime. Re-read it and then refocus yourself so you have your eye on the end result of your detoxing.

- **When you're eating, just eat.** This means that you shouldn't be eating in front of the TV. You shouldn't be listening to music while you eat. You shouldn't be reading while you eat. The main idea is to focus on you're eating and be mindful of it.

- **Don't stress over buying the exact same food items.** Most people stir clear of eating top quality foods like grass-fed or organic because their budget doesn't allow them to do so. Don't stress over this and find a way around it.

- **Replace the bad with the good when you're feelings are knocking on the door.** Emotions cannot be controlled and sometimes, or maybe most of the time, they overpower the will. This is why a lot of people drink, smoke or eat when they're feeling a lot of feelings brewing up.

  Don't make it difficult for yourself! I'm not saying that you should give in to the craving. What I mean is replace it with something healthy. For example, if you're a stress eater, you may want to have pre-prepared healthy snacks close by (*granted, of course, that they are included in your meal planning and daily calorie requirement*).

- **Preparation, Preparation, Preparation.** Remember to do your grocery shopping before the week begins. You may also prepare your ingredients ahead of time. You can do the chopping and the marinating for example.

- **Don't quit because you slipped the first time.** Ok so this is the difficult part. What if you slip? Chances are you will the first time but do not give up. Get back up, start again and focus more on the positive.

- **Last but not the least: Rest well. Exercise. Enjoy the outdoors and go play.** This is very self-explanatory. You're taking care of your body during the sugar detox, right? Don't limit yourself to just eating well. You also need to give your body the rest it need. On top of that, you need to distress by exercising or just having fun. Go out, see the world and put your phone down. Adapt an active lifestyle is what I'm saying.

Chapter 10

WORDS FROM THE AUTHOR

I just want to cease this moment to tell you that you're going to make it! As I said before, picking up this book was a good choice. The road that leads to a sugar free existence is paved with many obstacles but I'm telling you that you will make it until the end and you'll come out feeling and looking better than ever!

Don't just stick to this plan or this guide. Make it into your own; customize it to fit your preference. Journal your heart out. Seek for more knowledge online. Drink enough water. Exercise every day.

This is going to be your achievement. I know you can do it!

Chapter 11

BONUS – Sugar Free Dessert Recipes

I wanted to give you a bonus because I know that you're going to do such a good job in sticking with this detox so I've compiled 10 more sugar free dessert recipes to complete your meal planning. I don't want you to feel deprived even if you are snacking so here you go:

1. Cherries with Ricotta and Toasted Almonds

Calories per Serving	Prep Time	Total Time	Yields
150	10 mins	10 mins	1 Serving

Ingredients:

3/4 cup frozen pitted cherries

2 tablespoons non-fat ricotta

1 tablespoon toasted slivered almonds

Directions:

1. Heat cherries in the microwave on HIGH until warm, 1 to 2 minutes. Top the cherries with ricotta and almonds.

2. Sugar Free Lemon Cheesecake Mousse

Calories per Serving	Prep Time	Total Time	Yields
277	10 mins	10 mins	5 Servings

Ingredients:

8 ounces mascarpone cheese or cream cheese
1/4 cup lemon juice or 2 lemons
1 cup heavy cream
1/2-1 teaspoon lemon liquid stevia
1/8 teaspoon salt

Directions:

1. Add cream cheese and lemon juice to a stand mixer and blend until smooth.
2. Add heavy cream and the rest of the ingredients and blend until whipped.
3. Taste and adjust sweetener if needed.
4. Pipe into serving glasses and sprinkle on lemon zest if desired.
5. Keep refrigerated until ready to serve.

3. Sugar-Free Red Velvet Couple's Mug Cake

Calories per Serving	Prep Time	Cook Time	Yields
187	5 mins	3 mins	2 Servings

Ingredients:

1 tablespoon ground flaxseed

2 tablespoons coconut flour

1 tablespoon unsweetened cocoa powder

1/8 teaspoon sea salt

1/2 teaspoon baking pwoder

1/4 cup heavy cream

2 eggs

1/4 teaspoon vanilla extract

1 teaspoon cherry vanilla liquid stevia or vanilla stevia

Few drops red food coloring

Directions:

1. Whisk the first 4 ingredients together in a small bowl.
2. Whisk the rest of the ingredients together in another bowl.
3. Add the wet to the dry and stir until combined well.
4. Grease two 5 ounce ramekins and spread batter evenly into both.

5. Cook one at a time, in microwave for 1 1/2 minutes each.

6. Cool then frost as desired.

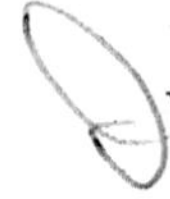

Vanilla Cream Cheese Frosting: No Sugar Added (Frosting for the Red Velvet)

Calories per Serving	Prep Time	Total Time	Yields
31	5 mins	5 mins	28 Servings

Ingredients:

1 1/2 cups cream cheese, lite

1 teaspoon vanilla extract

1 teaspoon vanilla stevia liquid

3 tablespoons heavy cream

Directions:

1. Using a stand mixer, place cream cheese, vanilla and stevia and mix until incorporated.

2. Add one tablespoon of heavy cream at a time until a smooth consistency appears.

3. Spoon into a pastry bag or plastic bag with a snipped corner to decorate or simply spread onto cake or cupcakes with a butter knife.

4. Keep refrigerated.

4. CocoNUT Bananas

Calories per Serving	Prep Time	Total Time	Yields
80	10 mins	10 mins	4 Servings

Ingredients:

4 teaspoons cocoa powder

4 teaspoons toasted unsweetened coconut

2 small bananas

Directions:

1. Place cocoa and coconut on separate plates.
2. Roll each banana slice in the cocoa, shake off the excess then dip in the coconut.
3. Spoon into a pastry bag or plastic bag with a snipped corner to decorate or simply spread onto cake or cupcakes with a butter knife.
5. Keep refrigerated.

5. Low Carb White Chocolate Coconut Fudge

Calories per Serving	Prep Time	Cook Time	Yields
175	5 mins	5 mins	24 Servings

Ingredients:

4 ounces cacao butter

1 can (15 ounce) coconut milk

1/2 cup coconut oil

1 cup coconut butter

1/2 cup vanilla protein powder

1 teaspoon vanilla extract

1 teaspoon coconut liquid stevia

A pinch of salt

Optional topping: unsweetened coconut flakes

Directions:

1. Melt the cacao butter in a sauce pan over low heat.
2. Stir in the coconut milk, coconut oil and coconut butter.
3. Continue to stir until completely smooth, no lumps.
4. Turn off heat and whisk is protein powder, vanilla extract , stevia and salt.

5. Pour mixture into a parchment lined 8 by 8 pan.
6. Sprinkle with coconut flakes if desired.
7. Refrigerate 4 hours or overnight.
8. Does not need to be kept refrigerated for storage.

6. Melon & Apple Granita

Calories per Serving	Prep Time	Cook Time	Yields
66	10 mins	4 Hours (Including Freezing Time)	8 Servings

Ingredients:

4 cups cubed ripe melon

1 cup unsweetened apple juice

1/4 cup lime juice

1 cup fresh blueberries

1 cup fresh raspberries

Fresh mint leaves, for garnish

Directions:

1. 13-inch glass or metal pan.

2. Place the pan on a level surface in your freezer. Freeze, stirring and scraping with a fork every 30 minutes, moving the frozen edges in toward the slushy center and crushing any lumps, until the granita is firm but not frozen solid, 3 to 4 hours.

3. Remove from the freezer; use a metal spatula or large spoon to break up the frozen ice into small slivers. Pack into an airtight plastic container and freeze for at least 1 hour more.

4. Remove from the freezer about 20 minutes before serving to soften slightly. Use a wide spoon or ice cream scoop to scrape the granita into shallow bowls. Sprinkle blueberries and raspberries over each portion and garnish with mint leaves, if desired.

7. Frosted Grapes

Calories per Serving	Prep Time	Cook Time	Yields
55	5 mins	50 mins (Including Freezing Time)	4 Servings

Ingredients:

2 cups seedless grapes

Directions:

1. Wash and pat dry grapes.
2. Freeze for 45 minutes.
3. Let stand for 2 minutes at room temperature before serving.
4. Enjoy during summer or enjoy during a hot day!

NOTE: You can also do this with other fruit.

8. Peanut Butter Ice Cream Sandwiches

Calories per Serving	Prep Time	Cook Time	Yields
124	5 mins	30 mins (Including Freezing Time)	8 Servings

Ingredients:

3 tablespoons no-sugar-added creamy peanut butter

2 cups vanilla no-sugar-added, fat-free ice cream, softened

16 (2-inch-diameter) gingersnaps

Directions:

Swirl peanut butter into ice cream. Place in freezer 30 minutes or until firm enough to spread.

Spread 1/4 cup ice cream mixture onto each of 8 gingersnaps. Top with remaining 8 gingersnaps. Place sandwiches on a 15-

x 10-inch jelly-roll pan; freeze until firm. Wrap sandwiches in plastic wrap, and store in freezer.

NOTE: To soften ice cream in the microwave, remove top and liner (if any) of carton. Microwave on HIGH (power level 10) in 10-second intervals, checking in between, until ice cream reaches desired consistency.

9. Chocolate Popcorn Bark

Calories per Serving	Prep Time	Cook Time	Yields
91	10 mins	60 mins (Including refrigeration)	18 Servings

Ingredients:

6 cups CVS ABound Light Popcorn

4 (1 ounce) packages CVS Abound Superfruit Baobab fruit bites

9 ounces Lily's Sugar-Free Chocolate Chips

Directions:

1. In a large bowl combine popcorn and 3 packages of Babao bites.

2. Melt chocolate chips for 1 minute in the microwave or heat in a small pot on the stove over low heat. Stir until smooth.
3. Line a baking pan with parchment paper.
4. Pour the melted chocolate over the popcorn and fruit bites.
5. Toss until well coated then lay close together on the baking pan. Sprinkle the last package of the Babao bites over the popcorn for color.
6. Refrigerate for one hour then break into pieces and serve in paper cupcake liners.

10. Chocolate Popcorn Bark

Calories per Serving	Prep Time	Cook Time	Yields
77	10 mins	40 mins	3 Dozen cookies

Ingredients:

2 cups uncooked regular oats

1 cup raisins

1 cup chopped walnuts

1/2 teaspoon salt

1 1/2 cups mashed banana (about 3 medium)

1/3 cup vegetable oil

1 teaspoon vanilla extract

Directions:

1. Preheat oven to 350°.
2. Combine first 4 ingredients in a large bowl; stir well. Combine banana, oil, and vanilla; stir well. Add banana mixture to dry ingredients, stirring to combine. Let stand 15 minutes.
3. Drop dough by rounded tablespoonfuls onto ungreased baking sheets. Bake at 350° for 15 minutes or until lightly golden. Transfer cookies to wire racks; cool completely. Refrigerate for one hour then break into pieces and serve in paper cupcake liners.

FAQ

Is this guide right for me?

Yes, if you would like to eliminate sugar in your diet. If you're a vegetarian or a vegan, you might need to stir away from other recipes but, generally, if you're a person who wants to be healthy by the elimination of sugar, then YES.

Will this guide be safe if I'm athletic?

If you have high activity levels, you have to make sure that you eat right and drink plenty of water. Use the guide on the prep phase checklist to see your daily calorie requirement and then go from there. As long as you remember to adjust your eating and drinking to your activity (*plus you avoid starving yourself*), yes it'll be alright for you to sugar detox while maintaining your active lifestyle.

Is this guide safe for diabetics?

Yes it is. All recipes in this guide are either sugar free or they have natural sugars in them. But, it's always a good idea to consult a doctor or a medical professional before taking on this sugar detox guide.

Can my family join in on this program?

Yes! In fact, it would be great if you're entire family could join in. That way, you wouldn't have to face the challenging obstacle of watching them eat whatever you're avoiding. The recipes are definitely fit for each member of the family.

Can I customize the meal plans?

Yes, like what we talked about earlier. It would be better if you put your personal touch into this so you'll have higher chances of becoming successful. By all means, research online for vegetable recipes that you can replace the meat recipes with if you're a vegetarian. You can add desserts to all of your meal plans. It's up to you. This guide was designed to be flexible and customizable so feel free.

Is it better if I pair my sugar detox with exercise?

Of course it is! The one thing that you have to remember, though, is you have to take it slow especially if you're activity level was sedentary. It's easy to get hyped up during the first weeks of sugar detoxing so many people will have the tendency to exercise excessively during this time. Remember that, during the first week, your body will slowly adjust so you have to expect sugar withdrawal effects like headaches and mood swings.

Do I start from Day 1 if I fell off the Wagon?

No. Go ahead and continue the plan at the point you're at. There's no need to go back to day 1. Anyway, remember that this will most likely be the first of many detoxes so just continue chugging along even if you had a small slip.

Hey,

If you liked this book, them I'm happy ☺

My hope is that it helped you in some way.

If you'd like to learn more about my other books, check out the info below:

Unleash the Power of the Paleo Diet

http://www.amazon.com/dp/B00VAMI5PY

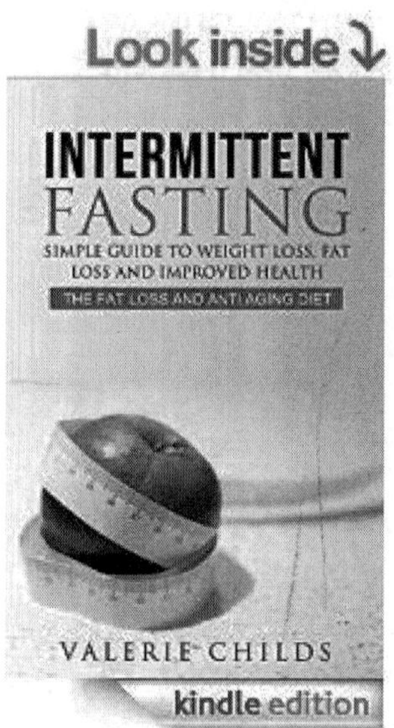

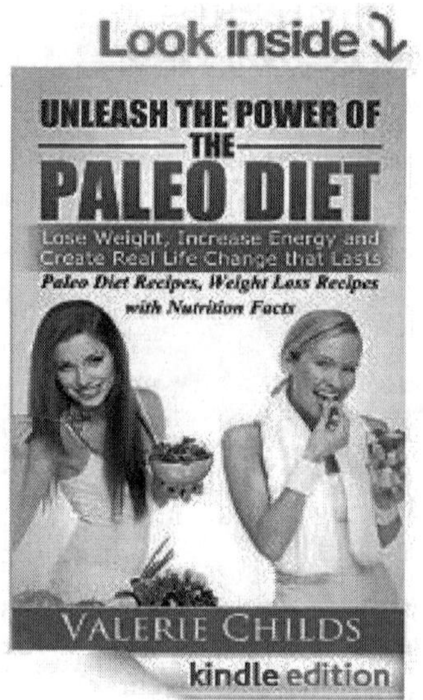

Intermittent Fasting

http://www.amazon.com/dp/B00VVC6O4W

Conclusion

Thank you again for downloading this book!

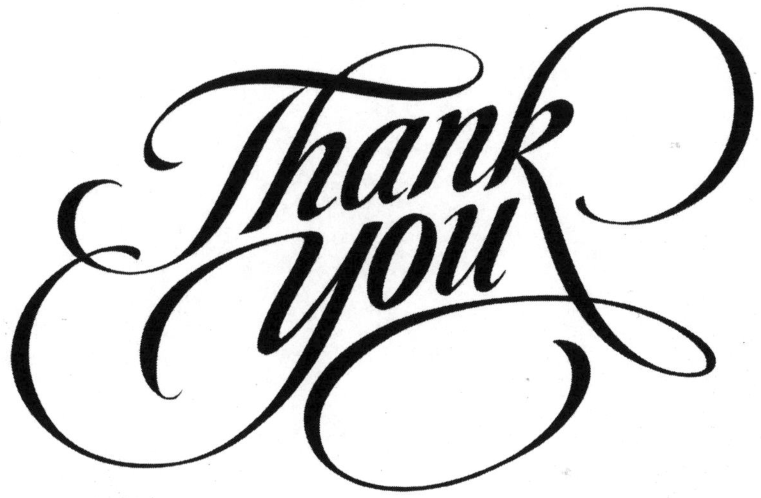

If you enjoyed this book, then I'd like to ask you for a favor, would you be kind enough to leave a review for this book on Amazon? It'd be greatly appreciated!

Help us better serve you by sending questions or comments to greatreadspublishing@gmail.com - Thank you!

Made in the USA
Middletown, DE
16 July 2015